The

Of Who We Are

A Guide To Understanding Who We Are:
Body, Heart, Spirit & Soul

MW00721196

INSTRUCTOR & HOLISTIC PRACTITIONER

KIMBERLEY ANNE BUCKLER

Copyright © 2015 by Kimberley Buckler

All rights reserved.

No part of this publication may be reproduced, distributed, or transmitted in any form or by any means, including photocopying, recording, or other electronic or mechanical methods, without the prior written permission of the publisher, except in the case of brief quotations embodied in critical reviews and certain other noncommercial uses permitted by copyright law.

Wholesale discounts for book orders are available through Ingram Distributors.

ISBN
978-1-987985-68-9 (softcover)
978-1-987985-67-2 (ebook)

Published in Canada.

First Edition

Table of Contents

Introduction

· ·

AFTER 40 YEARS OF EXPERIENCES I WAS DRAWN TO WRITING A book about the spirit realm.

My name is Kimberley Anne, and I was born and raised in Canada. My father was Australian and my mother was Canadian of European descent. My dad came to Canada in 1958 and met my mom around 1959. Both my brother and I were raised in Calgary Alberta.

This book has been written to help those who are learning that there is more than just human and animal's co-existing on this planet. For over a year I have wanted to promote a new healing technique, but something just came into play that told me it was time. I am also a Reiki Master / Intuitive that has been practicing for over 12 years with clients and teaching classes. Along with providing sessions for: Reiki, Intuitive Readings, Reflexology, Past Life Regression, House Clearings and Ear Candling, I teach Reiki, Building Your Intuition, and Crystal Healing. My fascination with holistic healing has led me down many paths and to go within to access the ancient healings.

Now my story will begin and I hope to help others to understand that: no, you are not crazy and the spirit realm is here. Blessings for your journey!

Dedication
·

THIS BOOK IS DEDICATED TO ALL THOSE ON THIS BEAUTIFUL planet that have at one time been labeled as not being normal. For those of us who see spirits and hear spirits. We may have been diagnosed as having multiple personalities, ADD, Autism, or Schizophrenia. Some of us are Indigos and Crystal children, who are sensitive/empaths. Not normal, is what we may hear. Many of us are put on medications instead of getting the help or support that they really need. This book is for us!

I would also like to dedicate this book to those who supported me while writing it and especially those who pre-read the book and provided encouraging feedback.

Also a huge hug and much love for my family and extended family who watched me go down this path, lovingly or with skeptical concerns.

Blessings to all and know within each of us is a beautiful soul waiting to be recognized!

Chapter 1

My Story

AUGUST 2, 2013 (A 7 DAY) I WOKE UP AT 3 A.M. AND COULD NOT get back to sleep. I had been dreaming of someone from 10 years ago. The dream was not nice. It was invasive. I turned on the computer. I don't normally do this when I am woken up by energy and spirits from within the dream state. In the dream I did know that others (light beings / angels) were looking after me. I had this weird urge to sit and write. I got the pencil and paper in my hand and was ready to write. I wrote a couple of words, but it did not feel right so I turned on the computer and started typing. I did not question anything and started typing the following:

I can feel my spirit guide at the top of my head. My ears were buzzing.

I asked: "What do you want me to share?"

The reply was: "We want you to listen: we want to help"

I asked again: "How?"

Reply: "Channelling."

Was wondering who this spirit being was. I asked: "Who are you?"

"Paladies."

I asked: "Who in Paladies?"

"The Counsel"

Me: "How can I help?"

"Relaying messages."

Asked: "What do you want to share?"

Reply "Trouble"

"How?"

"Infiltration of the dead"

"How can this be? Will each person be meeting their demons? Such as the spirits and I working together?"

Answer: "Yes."

"Is this world wide?"

"Yes."

"Fear?"

"Yes."

I asked "Please share what you would love me to say".

"God has given each of us a gift. Our gifts are our strength to work in the light. Our gifts allow us to shine, and continue shining. We can't stop to wonder. We just need to embrace what we love doing each time we feel that we are being challenged. In time we go to our heart centre we need to remember the love and light there and become that light. Don't allow yourself to get distracted by what others are thinking. Embrace that light. Continue the project till your vibration gets stronger and you feel that giddiness. That love. Send the divine blessings to those around you from the heart. We can all do this. The vibration of the blessings is filled with unconditional love, the love of the ascended masters and God / Creator. Ask your people to practice sending creator blessings. Tell them to embrace the energy of the ancient ones. These are the ones that truly helped to create the divine universe with the Creator. This source of love is strong. This love of source is the light you work with. End. "

I said: "Thank you."

Last comment "Blessings to all."

For this to all unfold and for me to lead up to how we can help out, I am going to tell you a story about parts of my life that brought me to this book.

In 1960 I was brought to 2 amazing souls, my mom and dad. Their love for each other was very strong, and they later had a son, my brother, who is just over a year younger than me. We were both their pride and joy. We were born in Calgary, Alberta and spent the first few years of our lives in the Kensington area.

I remember my brother and I both having bad dreams and waking Mom and Dad up because we were crying in our sleep. These dreams happened at the same time, as both of our beds were in the same room. One time that stood out, we were about 4 and 5 years old. In the morning my mom and dad were standing together, and Dad asked us what we were dreaming about the night before. They were quite concerned as we were both crying in our sleep and scared to go back to bed. After I had told my dad about my dream, my brother got quite mad at me and said that was his dream. This was just the start for me of working with those that are in the spirit form from the spirit realm. These types of scary dreams still continue.

The dreams could be of getting hurt, helping others, escaping, spirits and so much that I still don't remember in the morning. My brother and I continued to have bad dreams at the same time, and this also happened with my youngest daughter and I.

I have memories of energies in different houses that we lived in. The bad dreams started in a house on Kensington Road in Calgary around the age of 5 or earlier. We lived in several houses as children, some okay and some with weird experiences. The next house that scared me was in Vancouver, British Columbia in the Capillano area. I had bad dreams of the furnace room in that house and swore there was someone buried under the cement floor. This dream was a repeated dream that I had, in which my brother and I knew someone was buried in the furnace room, but we were scared to tell anyone. In the dream, we had to be quiet about the body. Once in a while I would even have this same dream about the same house in other places that we lived in. These dreams were of spirits and dead bodies.

When we first moved to Vancouver, my mom was really sick and my brother started walking in his sleep. We knew we had to keep ourselves busy and give mom time to rest. I started to know things that were not voiced, but I knew the truth. I remember my dad confronting me one day and asking me why I said something to my brother about mom. My statement was, "I had to Dad, no one was telling him the truth." I knew things, but not knowing why or how.

About this time, I started day dreaming about saving the world and people around me. I was about 7 years old. At school, I would stand in the playground and day dream during recess and lunch. I dreamt of ways I could save the world or stick up for my brother.

Other days I did play, marbles, skipping, but was not asked to all that often, as I was pretty shy and even at that time the kids were not very friendly. One time on the way home, I ended up beating up a boy my age that was picking on my brother, and I had to stop myself before I really hurt him. This group of kids never bothered us again, but I was later ashamed of hurting someone. My dad taught us never to hurt first, only to defend ourselves. This was a time when I was really scared for my brother and did not want him to be hurt.

The reason that I shared the story about sticking up for my brother, was that hearing someone be insulted or teased always bothered me, even as a child. I would feel their embarrassment and shame. I felt bad for the one being picked on. To me this bantering was not funny, and I then realized how sensitive I was. Later I found out this was about being empathic, physically and emotionally. I never felt like I fit in.

The next house that I had spirit adventures in was in Southwood, Calgary Alberta. I was about 11 years old. Teen age hormones were already starting to kick in. My body was changing, and I started to feel the presence of my spirit guide. I don't know what time it was, but just as I was falling asleep, I would feel jolt at the back of my neck area and heard an electrical sound zing through my head. I found out much later that my brother experienced this same thing at night. Whenever this happened, it would always scare the day lights out of me, as I was just about to drift off to sleep. I would be zapped awake again.

In this house I would wake up at night scared to death. Some nights when I woke up I could see spirits all around my bed. I saw the faces. Some were scary and some were not. But what really scared me was what we call entities. I never saw the entities, and they always hurt me, by poking me hard. The pain was there in the dream state and when I was semi-conscious during the dream. The entities were always closer to the floor and reached up to get me. This, along with the feeling of being held down in a paralyzed state became a trend for what I called my bad dreams, later known as spirit dreams.

These dreams started to happen no matter where I lived after that. The next house that I lived in, with my Dad and my brother, was in another area in Southwest Calgary. But this house had something in the wall in my bedroom. I remember always trying to cover my head at night, trying to protect myself. Just about 5 years ago (2010), a Shaman friend saw me in this house and saw the wall beings. I believe these to be spirits that were stuck in the house and they seemed to gather by my bed at night. I would try to read as long as I could at night, dreading having to go to sleep. Sleep time there was not very peaceful at all.

This was about the time my grandmother started to mention my bad dreams. She thought it all had to do with my step mother who used to abuse my brother and I. Nan was quite concerned as I was scared even during the day and could not deal with loud noises. I had a troubled teen age life, not knowing what was bothering me and why I was so sensitive. Not into makeup, fancy clothes and idle gossip, I spent more time with my brother and his friends. As this was going on, I believe that I started lucid dreaming and learning how to fly in my dreams. I was running from trouble in the dreams, helping others, dreaming of spirits and more. Sometimes we were looking for hidden escape routes, which I now believe to be past life experiences.

Around this time I started to have dreams of old houses with long hallways, ghosts and antique furniture. Sometimes the furniture was given to me, or I knew whose it was. The hallways scared me, as I could see the shadows of the ghosts /spirits going from room to room. The antique furniture always seemed to have significance, but I did not know why. Many of the old houses in the dreams were boarding houses, with many bedrooms, monsters, and spirits and I was scared of the unknown. I think some of them were hotels or houses of past relatives.

During my troubled teens I ran away a lot, but always knew what was legally right or wrong. I saw kids taking heroin for the first time and walked away. I watch other people steal, and wreck things around them. I watched young ladies get drawn into prostitution. Each time I saw this stuff I would always able to say no and stay on the good side of the law. I rarely drank alcohol and knew that the street life was dangerous.

I had premonitions that made me feel queasy. When I did not follow them, I always found out why I had felt uneasy. One premonition happened before going out with a friend. I remember thinking, *Kimmy, don't be a chicken. Just go.* The driver of the van ran dead centre into a tree. The roads were snowy and icy. That was the end of that evening out.

By the time I was 14 or 15 I had had a profound vision that kept me alive. This vision showed me a bit of what was to come into my life. In the vision I saw a fellow, over 30 years old, gruff, like a mountain/ country person and I knew that I had children. This vision saved my life and I knew then that I was needed by my future children.

When I was from 14 – 16, I lived at the YWCA in Lethbridge, Alberta. I was still the troubled teen. My best friend was a native gal that introduced me to life in the reserves west of Lethbridge.

I got to go to the pow wows, learnt how to properly enter a tee pee, went to volley ball tournaments and started to learn some beading. During this time I also learnt the name of white women spoken in the native language. I knew when I was being talked about. But this did not matter, as when I was out in the native community I felt like I was at home. There was no materialistic living there and life seemed so much more laid back. I knew that things were not always easy on the reserve, but it was a community where everyone looked out for each other.

During this time, I had another profound vision. In the dream, I was flying towards a teepee. There was a man and woman standing in front of the teepee and a huge brown bear standing to the side. This image stayed with me for years. Later on when I started to get involved in natural healing, I found out that my spirit guide was a medicine man.

As I grew into an adult, I was learning about better eating patterns. I did gain a couple of friends. I always seemed to be on guard and not very trusting. I still had more male friends as they were not catty, into make-up and fancy clothes. They did not gossip and seemed to be more grounded. During this time I was very careful how I did things and always concerned about my health.

I was almost 22 when my first child was born and almost 24 when my second child joined us. Each one of them brought many experiences and many questions were answered later on. My love for both of these little ones was strong, and I knew they were meant to be with me. This was part of the vision I had when I was 14. The oldest always knew when I was troubled about something and hovered around me till I settled down or if I was sick. I was always very discreet about what was bothering me. The youngest always seemed to have bad dreams when I did. I would wake up from my bad dream and I would hear the little one crying out in the dream state. I would go into their room and gently bring the little one out of the dream.

When the children were 2 years old and the other 2 months old we moved into a town house in Southwest Calgary. At night time, I would hear footsteps go down the hallway when the kids were in bed. It was like a spirit would check up on them. I never did see the spirit but would always hear the bedroom door open then close. I later found out that there was a huge blood stain on the carpet by the back door when the previous tenants had moved out. There was a patch of new carpet when we moved in. My children also told me of an older man spirit that they saw there, it would hide under the stairs in the basement. After moving out I would have dreams of scary spirits that lived there. The dreams were always unsettling.

When I lived in the town house, I started to vision living in a home with a huge yard and many gardens. I would dream about flying towards the hills/mountains for safety. In the dream I would see the natives living on the south side of the river, and that area represented gardening and safety. I also wanted to move to Cochrane, Alberta, as I loved the town, but was scared to be too far away from the doctors while the girls were small. By the time they were 2 and 4, I was a single parent and doing the best I could. I went to SAIT (the Southern Alberta Institute of Technology) to take accounting and business administration for 2 years. But at that time, I knew it would never be right for me to work for a big company or corporation.

When the kids were 9 and 11 we moved to Cochrane. After a bit I realized I was where I was meant to be for the next phase of life. The dreams of flying into the safety of the hills stopped. I met up with who became my second husband. At this time, we were very much into eating well, cooking healthy food, and learning to preserve food for the winter. From the time my oldest child was a baby I had learnt about living in a heathy environment with healthier cleaning products. During this time I had also found out how sensitive I was to chemicals too.

As my children were into their teen age years and working in a family-based construction company, the stress had me looking into vitamin B complex to help. At this time, my husband introduced me to a natural healer. This introduction was the beginning of connecting the dots. I started to learn more about energy healing (which I was unknowingly doing when my oldest child was a baby with colic.)

After taking a couple of workshops with this new friend and healer, along with some treatments, a new world started to open up. I was told to read a book that brought a profound message *"The Eagle and the Rose"* by Rosemary Altea. This book was a start into a new journey and understanding what natural healing was about. I learnt that yes, energy work is very powerful, and yes, working with the spirit realm is okay. Right after reading this book in 2 days I went to see the local psychic. She shared with me that I was a powerful psychic and healer, and when the doubt showed on my face, she called in the healer that I had been working with to confirm this. I was shocked, humbled and scared.

On the way home, after hearing what the psychic shared, I started to hyperventilate and had to sit down on the curb for a while till I could breathe again. What I felt was fear coming in. Was I safe? Could I really be who this lady said I was? Then memories of this life time started to come to mind. About this time, I was close to 40 years old. This is the age when many females start into the crone state. With years of experiences and with children nearly grown up, I had gathered a lot of knowledge. With this the next journey started.

I just got a reminder from my spirit guide to share how I realized what the electrical zinging was that I have felt at night since I was a kid. When I was talking to the psychic, I asked how we do energy work. She said just to go home, find a quiet spot and start. Well, I went home, thought of someone that I would like to help, and asked for the energy to flow through really strong for this person. I heard and felt that electrical zing over and over. I was shocked and nervously laughed. Then I realized this was what I had been feeling and hearing for so many years before going to sleep. This was the beginning of learning to connect the dots for my experiences. This was the start of really becoming in tune with my true self. Along with this new experience, I was learning that my spirit guide had a good sense of humour too. We started to work together as a team.

I need to share a bit more before we really start with the rest of this guide book.

From the year 2000 (I had turned 40) to the year 2002, I started to learn how to do card readings for others and got my Reiki Master certificate. With the readings, I was learning really quickly how to listen to what I was hearing and realized that my knowing was very strong. I just needed the time to learn and to trust what I was hearing, feeling, and knowing. The instructor that was teaching the psychic workshop realized what was going on for me, and that I was a quick learner. I was dismissed from the workshop very quickly as she was intimidated by me somehow, even though I was really quiet. I was crushed, but after a bit I knew I needed to learn this on my own. With the Reiki workshops that I took, I learnt a lot more on how we can energetically heal others around us along with healing our bodies. The Reiki also helped me to open more to the spirit realm and strengthen my psychic skills.

Over time I started to ask my spirit guide and the universe to teach me how to tap into mediumship (I do this more through the Reiki sessions for clients), how to pick up on animal spirits around people, and how to learn with the spirit realm. I wanted to be able to see the spirit realm again, but still needed to learn more. Around the year 2005 I started to do house clearings. During a house clearing we can use sage to cleanse a home of energies that were created by abuse, sickness and energy imprints. I also tap into the Reiki energy during these clearings to assist with the sage. Then we can use sweet-grass to bring in blessings for the home. In this time I also learnt about the angels and Arch-angels who are some of God's helpers. Archangel Michael helped me out a lot with the house clearings and feeling safe.

In 2007 I was brought 2 students/ friends that brought many experiences forth for me. With them I learnt more about the fairy realm. This is when the bottom of my legs would start to get cold to let me know that the fairies were there for clients. These new friends also taught me about scary spirits, and spirit that went dark. I was asked to smudge their home. I saw one of their spirit guides in a hologram like picture. I could see the spirit guides face. Then later, one of them came for a session, in which I was shown another dark spirit, then later she came for a session for walk-ins and a light body integration.

With all of this going on and along with all of the learning, I realized that I was on my true path. I was a healer, empath, and strong intuitive. My dreams about houses, antique furniture, and spirits stopped. I was doing what I was dreaming as a child, as I was learning how to work comfortably with the spirit realm.

Since 2006 I have been doing presentations for different groups on natural healing and sharing about the potential of energy work. Around 2009, I started to do workshops in smaller towns for Usui Reiki, Crystal Healing, and Building Your Intuition. With these presentations and workshops, I provided a lot of support for everyone that attended, no matter how much they already knew. We learn together in a community. During these events, I used my personal experiences as part of the teaching, to share that I had been there and was always open to learning more.

Over the last 4 years I have been learning more about who we are. In the past year, I have had 2 accidents that I thought set me back, but they were valuable lessons. This last accident showed me that it is time to step it up and share my experiences. Now, this guide book will go into some different areas to help those who are reading this learn more about what is going on around them.

Chapter 2

The Essence of Who We Truly Are

THIS CHAPTER WILL OPEN SOME DOORS FOR YOU. I DO NOT PRO-
claim to know it all, nor do I intend to offend anyone as this is
what I have experienced and learnt.

2012 (a 5 year, year of change) was a year of learning for me
on who we truly are. As a child I was introduced to the Anglican
faith but did not attend church for long. My dad shared with
me that we did have a personal angel with us. This I had forgot-
ten until I was older. When I was 12 years old, the step mother
tried to get me involved with the church again, and I was to go
through a confirmation. The teaching of the religion was that we
came from Adam and Eve. This did not make sense as there are
many races/nationalities. At the same time, school (science) was
teaching about man evolving from the apes. Of course teenage
hormones, mixed with some common sense that was still intact,
said that both were conflicting beliefs, and neither was very

believable. I proclaimed to be atheist for many years till I was about 35 years old, and then I realized that there was more to this big picture. In 2005 I was introduced to the angel realm through a workshop that I was guided to take. I have had other healers tell me I was an Earth angel. This information I humbly kept to myself, as I did not really believe it even then and was scared to share.

During this time came the understanding that there was a greater being: God, Creator, Spirit. This being was here for the highest good of all. It did not matter what we believed in, this amazing being was here to guide us and help us grow. This being did not judge, hate or fear. This being was pure divine love.

The angels and ascended masters are God's helpers from the angel realm, and some of them did live on this planet at one time in human form. Brother Jesus is one of our ascended masters! As I learnt more about the angels, I felt that we were never truly alone. We can receive a lot of messages from the angel realm and they are there to support us. Our guardian angels will never interfere, but they will assist, like when I had the profound vision when I was 14, the vision that showed me what was to come into my life. I have traveled many miles with the angels and have even felt them around me.

The animal spirits and fairies are also part of the other realms that are here to assist us. I will get more into this in Chapter 11.

In 2006 I learnt what it felt like to have divine intervention come into my energy field. When this happens for me I feel the love of God /Creator so strongly that I can have tears flowing down my face. This energy is very powerful! This can help us remember who we really are. When I share a blessing or prayer, and when the angels want to show their presence during a Reiki treatment for a client, the angel energy or divine love enters my whole being, and I cry happy tears.

In 2012, I had a Reiki student/friend use me as a practice client for a workshop that she was taking. At this time, I knew we were more than we were taught, but I was still not grasping it all to really understand. When she had gathered all her information together for me, she double checked with her instructor to make sure it was right. Her instructor confirmed what my friend had found out. I believe that she was able to access my Akashic Records. The Akashic Records are the history of our soul and are accessed psychically or through meditation.

The reason that I am sharing this now is that I have met more sisters and brothers with the same linage, and so feel more comfortable sharing this information and not in ego.

Before we go on, here are a few facts that have been supported by those in the holistic field but also by psychologists and scientists.

DNA testing can show:

1. We each have a blood lineage: this is proven through DNA testing. We can prove who our blood parents are. Even aunts, uncles and siblings share the same genetic DNA.

2. Through bloodlines, we can see recognizable traits, thought patterns and health discomforts or strengths.

Researchers of psychology and even doctors have shown:

1. Many of us have had more than one life on planet Earth.

2. We have a soul family, which is not always related by blood.

3. Many souls have come from other planets and galaxies. Edgar Cayce brought a lot of this information forward for us. There are many other well known researchers and scientists in the past and present that will back this up.

Now when we look at the bigger picture, we start to open doors to more understanding of who we really are. We all are a spark of God/Creator. We started off as pure divine light and love. We were directed to planets that needed us and planets where we could have experiences and lessons to help ourselves grow more and to be there to assist in other's experiences and growth.

We are back to who we really are.

Each one of us is a spark of God. Each of us has pure divine love and light within. Each of us has had or will have more than one life time here on Mother Earth. Each one of us is learning how a spiritual being can live in a human body in a 3-D existence.

Also there is life after death. I believe and know that we get the chance to evolve and grow more than one life time. I know that I have had many lives here as a healer in many different cultures. I know that I felt safer in the cultures where natural healing was accepted and part of the culture. I saw in past life regressions where I was a medicine man in Africa and Native America. I was a healer in India. In that life time I saw myself in a bright yellow shirt with a string of beads hanging from my neck. I was a male with twin boys and had a wife. In these lives I felt safe as this was part of the natural culture. In other life times, my body was hung or burnt, or I had to stay in hiding for my own safety. I was known as one who knew the truth. A truth seeker was someone to be careful around, as this person knew what was really going on and lies would be seen through. This term, "truth seeker" along with "Bringing Heaven to Earth." was something I was guided to put on my website. Then later on, I came to understand why.

Now to you!

When I have a client on the table for a healing session, or even when talking to a person, I have learnt how we can feel the true essence of your soul. The essence of your soul can show so much and provide a bit of history on what you have gone through. Depending on what needs to be brought forward for that time. The feeling I get from your soul is pure love. This love is so strong that I get tears in my eyes each time.

It does not matter where you have been, or what you have seen, done or accomplished: I still feel that strong creator love within you. You are a miracle and blessing that has managed to survive so far on this planet among such harsh conditions, ego, fear and judgment. You are a spark of God/Creator within. You are an amazing soul that got stuffed into a human body. Our light body / spirit can be much bigger than what we realize and have been led to believe.

This being said and shared, the feeling of love that I can feel within you is similar to love of the angel realm. I can see some of the healing that you are going through or will still need to go through. I want you to know that you are loved! You are amazing no matter what state of mind you are in. This same love I have also felt in the presence of a monk. I was shaken by the power and beauty of the love he held in his space. This too was a lesson for me.

Over the last few years I have tried to explain what true love is and have had a hard time expressing it properly. It seemed that I was alone, that no one could truly tap into this. Was I weird? Was I an alien? Who was I? Just as you are reading this book, I learnt who we really are. With feeling the energy of the angels, I found out what true love was.

As we go on, I will explain in the following chapters the things that I have highlighted. I will continue with the guidance of my spirit guide and my fellow light beings and angel helpers.

Chapter 3

· · · · · · · · · · · · · · · · · · ·

Our Light Body and Soul: The Evolution of Souls and Our Star Friends

WHEN WE ARE WORKING WITH CLIENTS, WHETHER PROVIDING readings or energy work we can connect to their spirit and soul like what was mentioned in Chapter 2. When the soul is strong and vibrant, the energy is amazing. This is pure love. When the soul has had a tough time, you can still feel the love, but it is much fainter. When someone does not love themselves for who they truly are, I am shown this love to share with them.

In 2013 I was brought many clients that were not original Earth souls, along with learning to work with walk-ins. This chapter will focus more on our star friends.

Now we need to go back to what I had learnt from my dear friend. She found out that I had started in the Arcturian area. Arcturus is in the Bootes constellation, 36 light years from planet Earth. This is where we learn to be fully in the heart centre. Unconditional love is taught. Also according to Edgar Cayce the Arcturian's are one of the most advanced civilizations in this galaxy. They also have the energy and experience to help others heal physically, emotionally, mentally and spiritually. Arcturus is also known as the gateway to death and rebirth.

A little more on the Arcturians: they can share how you can co-exist in the pure love that is known as God energy and unconditional love. They are quite telepathic, empathic, and extremely sensitive and can help spirits of human and animal souls pass over to the other side. They also work closely with the angels and what is known as the Brotherhood of all. They are also from a 6th or 7th dimension.

When souls from other planets or galaxies come here, many times they forget who they are, and where they started from. Many things may feel familiar, but the person may feel alone. Also, the human does not remember everything from life time to life time. These individuals may need the assistance of deep meditation, hypnotherapy and past life regression.

There are many other beautiful beings out in the universe/ heavens and on planet Earth known as Mother Earth or Gaia. Each of these beings has made tremendous contributions to humanity and the evolution of our sisters and brothers in other areas of the galaxy.

Back to what I wanted to share personally, hearing this information, was both honoring and exciting. But within I knew that I needed to be humble. To me this was an honour. After hearing this report from my friend and doing some clearing, some of my answers were being answered as to why I was drawn to the holistic field. In November of 2012, I was introduced to another healer that did channeling through Archangel Michael. Mark explained to me more about the evolution of souls (of which I will get into later). At the end of the reading he said that sometimes he could not look directly at a person's energy/soul, as the light was too bright. He was referring to the energy he was seeing around me. Again, I was surprised. This message was honoring and I knew I needed to be humble.

After this, I started to meet and recognize more star sisters and brothers, some from the same area and some from other galaxies. What an honor! What an adventure! This was an affirmation of other souls being here too.

Each planet or civilization has its own unique traits and gifts that are shared amongst the universe and to help their star sisters and brothers out. Some sister planets are very peaceful, some strong protectors and some very much into the healing arts. After I found out that I was from Arcturus, I started to see some friends from other planets show up.

As I went along, I heard about other planets like Pleiades, Lyran, Orion, and more. There are also beings such as the Etherians, Bernarians, Cetians (they work with the Pleiadeans), Dals, The Greens, Suvians, Hyadeans, Korendians (who claim to be working with the Arcturians), and Vegans. It appears that many of these beings could be quite friendly and have assisted on Earth at one time or another.

Then we have other beings that are not walking in the light. By this I mean, they operate for greed and control. They have no consciousness of what havoc is created by their actions and they want to take over, and not for the highest good of all. These beings are part of what has caused wars around the world. They don't take into account that we are all sisters and brothers, and they seem to have no concept of unconditional love/God/Creator.

In 2013, I met the first fellow friend, from another planet, who is an amazing soul and very strong in personality. He is a very old soul and spoke of his home no longer being here. His planet had disappeared hundreds of years ago and he has helped out on this planet for almost as long, sometimes in human form, and sometimes as a spirit guide. At first, I was not sure as his stories were startling, but they were consistent. He also helped me to understand a lot of what I was learning and about the different energies.

In the summer of 2013, I started to get clients that were what I call walk-ins. We will revisit that in the next chapter. These were all very strong souls that were here again to help out. As I got more comfortable knowing that "Alien energy was walking among us", more doors opened and questions were once again being answered. As I started to look at those who were in my circle of friends, I realized that I was not alone. When I shared with clients and close friends what I was learning, they felt comfortable enough to share more about their theories and what they had encountered.

In 2014 I started to see the true essence of the planets that some clients are from. With the first person when I saw his original shape from his home land I was taken back. He felt like a warrior. Then I started to get images/visions of his body armour. He also appeared to have a bird like structure, similar but different from the human form. And he had a huge wing span. When I shared this information with him, he said that the Reiki practitioner that he usually went to saw the same thing. I believe this fellow was from the Vega region.

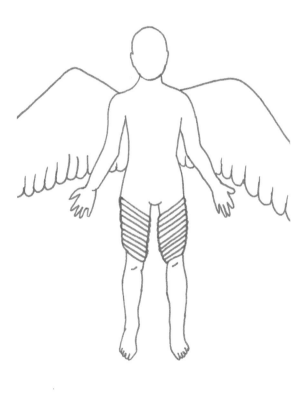

About a month later I was doing long-distance healing for my brother who lives in Australia. When I energetically had him on the healing table I saw metal bands on his arm. These metal bands that I saw were not of the Earth plane. They were created with a metal and constructed in a way that I have not seen here on Earth.

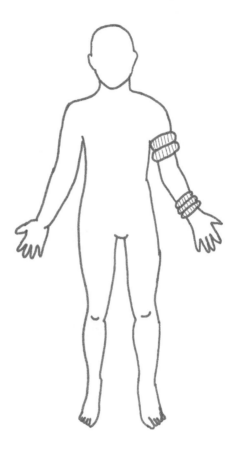

After this I started to see in more detail the wings of some clients. While working with one friend, I asked where fairy wings were located on a fairy's back, mischievously, I was holding back on what I saw. Right away she pointed to the middle of her back, and said "There." She was very serious and definite with her answer. When I chuckled, she looked at me funny, and I explained what I saw. With this, she shared how many times other people said that she had fairy energy about her. Then she started to giggle, realizing what she had shown me. It all started to sink in for her.

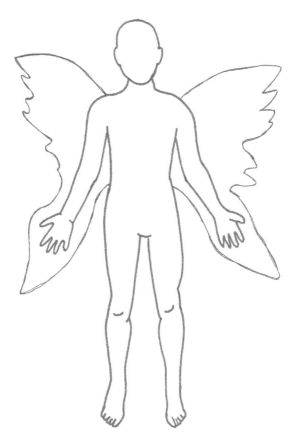

As time went on, I came to the realization that we are more than what we seem or are taught to believe. Many souls are from other planets, and I truly believe that each nationality came from a different region of the galaxy, hence different body structures, energies and skull formations.

I have a dear friend that introduced me to the ancient crystal skulls. These skulls were brought here hundreds, maybe thousands of years ago. When I first saw the 2 skulls that he had, I looked at the smaller skull and knew it was from a healer. The other one was a master's skull. How did I know this? It just came to me, and after doing some research, I got the affirmations on my first impressions. There are not many of the ancient crystal skulls, and most of them are in personal homes being looked after. When you see one of the ancient skulls you know it was not created with our technology. The 2 that I saw both had a rough surface to them, and the larger of the 2 still had dirt between the teeth. It had been buried a long time ago. This was mentioned as another sign of civilization here on Earth being much older than what we have been taught.

With this all being said, we will go to the evolution of our souls and our bodies.

When I met a fellow that did channeling, he shared some information through Archangel Michael.

Archangel Michael is here to help us in many ways, like all the angels of the light. He wanted me to know about the development of the souls:

Baby soul:

This soul that is just starting out. This soul is unconditionally loving and innocent

Young soul:

This soul may have gone through many life times and experiences. A young soul may also be one that is very power or money hungry. A young soul wants the most of everything, despite what it takes to reach that goal. Many times, the soul has to revisit the same lesson over and over till it realizes the lessons or ripple effect that it has created to achieve its goals. This soul needs to learn that it is not all about them.

Midterm soul:

A soul that is more concerned about religion, using force and protection.

Old soul:

A soul that has been down many roads and has had many life times on planet Earth. Along with this they have realized that things are not as they seem. Many can see beyond what is being presented. Many are becoming healers at this time to help opens the doors to spirituality and don't feel comfortable with organized religion and structured beliefs. This is not an easy phase even if one has evolved. The old soul has started to put the pieces together and usually is a very sensitive soul. These souls have the toughest time on this planet. They have learnt all that they need to know and start putting all their learnt information together. These souls you may find more into the healings arts.

So far we now know that our soul is more powerful than we have been taught. Not all souls are from planet Earth. We are all here together to help each other out and at this period of time, we are helping each other to walk away from fear and learn more about our true history. Like what was discussed in Chapter 2, our blood line is not necessarily our soul line.

When we walk and live in the heart centre our spirit shines brightly, as we are connected to our soul and God /Creator. Our body, spirit and soul radiate good health and wellbeing. We are here to work as a community and support all our sisters and brothers around the world.

Next we will visit our light bodies and human experiences.

Chapter 4
· · · · · · · · · · · · · · · · · ·

Our Light Body and the Effects of Human Experiences

OUR HUMAN BODY CONSISTS OF THREE MAJOR COMPONENTS: the physical body, the spirit and the soul. The spirit and soul of a person needs to be healthy, just like the physical body. I consider the spirit/soul part of the body as the light body or the energy body of our being. The soul is connected to the divine source, which is pure unconditional love and the vibration is high. The spirit is the energy of the soul that feels the emotions, sad and happy.

It is said that we are all spiritual beings having a human experience. It is hard for those who are highly evolved beings to live on the planet Earth and to watch all the distress, wars and pain. When the old souls or spiritual souls have done their work, it is easier to watch and observe.

The physical body:

The physical body is the vessel we need to live in while we are here on Mother Earth. It is more solid, having a physical shape with organs and blood encased within. With the physical body we need to be nourished properly so that emotional wellbeing of the body is healthy too. Vitamins, minerals, fibre, proper proteins, enzymes and oils are very important. When the physical body's needs are not met, we become sick physically, mentally and spiritually.

1. The physical body sick: sore shoulders, anger in the liver, heartbroken, sore elbow and knee. These areas appear as dark energy when I do a visual body scan. These areas can feel cold when I run my hands across the body.

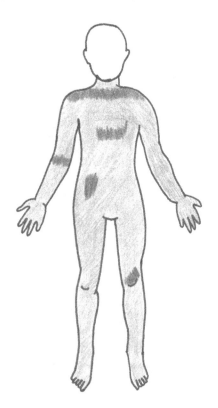

The light/spirit body:

The light /spirit body can be huge. It is bigger than the physical body and needs to extend beyond the physical form. This to me appears as light filaments, strands of bright light. The light/spirit and soul body are connected to the divine source, which is pure unconditional love and the vibration is high. One may see this source as God, Creator, or Mother Earth. This source is what you would consider a higher being of love and light. In this higher source of light, there is no ego and no judgment, no fear or pain. It is pure beauty. It feels like being in heaven.

When the light body is fully engaged within a person, there is less chance of other energies trying to occupy our space, as the vibration is really high. If something is not of the light, it has a hard time existing in this field of energy.

In 2013 I met a new student that has become a mentor to me. He has been teaching me more about the spirit realm. He shared how the vibration of the energy we were bringing in with the Reiki and the light body integration was so strong, that another energy that was residing in his physical body space left. I will share this more in the next chapter on walk-ins. Thus, his vibration became so strong that he only felt his own presence, and life became more peaceful.

The physical and light body together:

When both the physical and light body blend together, there should be a high vibrating energy within and without. There should be no shadows, only glowing health on all levels, physically, mentally, emotionally and spiritually.

2. The physical and spiritual vibrating high: good health, energy flows freely

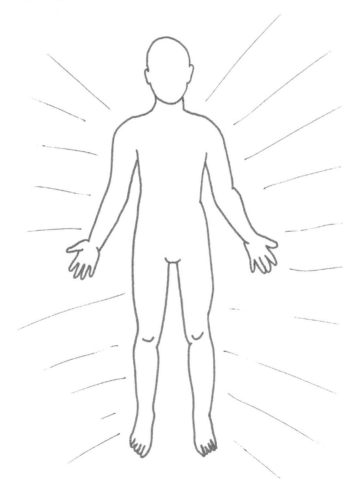

Life on planet earth can be hard, and those that come here are exposed to different emotions and

hard to deal with experiences: anger, fear, sadness, loss, judgement and many more emotions that are hard on the human body, mind and spirit. Light experiences such as happiness, love, and joy bring a light and gentle energy to the body, and the mind is joyful.

When we go from life time to life time we can accumulate a heavy load to carry. This happens when the soul /physical body holds onto fears, anger and resentment and has not been able to resolve or heal the past trauma in the life time in which it occurred.

Past traumas can be seen in many ways:

- The loss of a parent, sibling, spouse, friend or anyone that we became close to can create a trauma or leave behind sadness and regrets. It might have been someone that was there to help protect us when we felt down or un-supported in other ways.

- Physical and emotional abuse are also heavy energies that can create havoc in our lives and can create mental sickness and unease.

- Being attacked for who we are can create negative energies.

We will get more into this later on. Traumas can be carried from life time to life time. Or the traumas can go from parent to child to grandchild. When the soul has past experiences, the energies can be transmitted into the physical body. This is what I have seen with clients:

3. The physical body is clouded, the spirit of the body is low.

No energy is flowing at all. The person could be quite sick and depressed. All of the chakras are fully blocked.

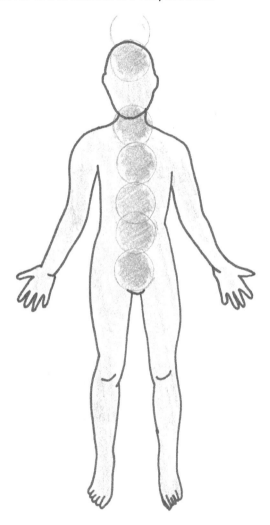

4. We can have a present life soul with trauma:

Holes appear to be blown through the grid and this shows me that a soul retrieval is required. The soul may need a lot of chakra clearing. I see the energetic grid around the body when a soul retrieval is needed. The grid appears about 2 feet above the body.

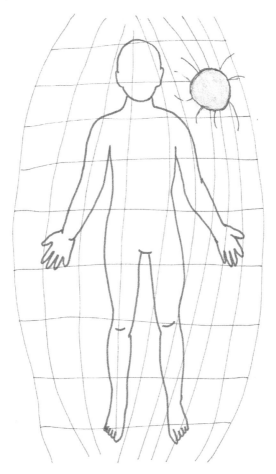

5. A soul with trauma:

A soul can have past-life imprints. These imprints appear to be shadows or blotches on the soul line.

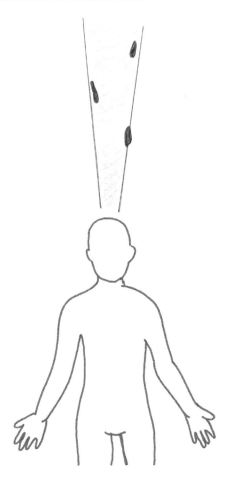

6. A spirit / soul that does not want to be seen,

This soul may have had past experiences that it may be ashamed of. Or something happened in a past life where this person had to hide who they were. (E.g. many psychics and healers hid during the dark times when there was burning and hanging of natural healers.)

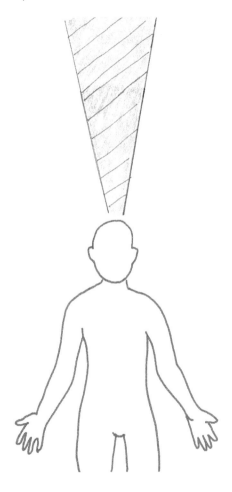

7. A spirit / soul that is clear, healthy, and has no imprints.

This person is happy and healthy on all levels.

As I work with clients I am shown the different situations either through a vision that I receive or a knowing of what happened. Sometimes, I am guided to ask a series of questions, but as I ask the questions, I get the whole picture. This then leads into healing of the physical, the spirit and the soul healing on all three levels.

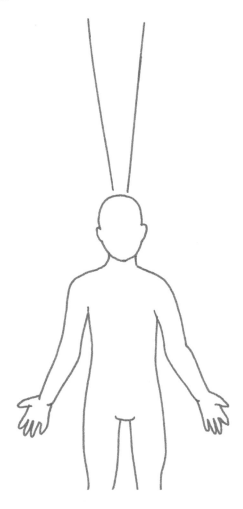

I got it! I keep seeing the number 3. When the body (physical), spirit and soul and balanced, we are in the state of divinity! I have seen the pattern of 3's. I have been guided to place three dots on the animal friends in my batiks and drawings.

As we go along on this amazing planet, we have had many experiences and also questions about why are things are happening. What can we do to change situations, our health and our thoughts? Why do I seem to be clouded or blocked? Why do I keep getting sick? Some of what is stated in this chapter and the next 2 chapters will lead to healing of the body on all three levels.

We have covered the essence of who we are, and our physical and light body and how trauma can appear. Now we are going to go a step further.

Chapter 5

. . . .

Walk-ins

IN 2013 I WAS INTRODUCED TO WALK-INS. IT WAS AS IF I KNEW who they were with only having a vague memory or hearing about them. A walk-in is when a human body has become a host for 2 souls for the life time of the body.

I will explain how this all started. In the summer of 2013, a lady that I had known of through another friend called to book a Reiki session with me. When she got here, she was sharing a bit about how she felt disconnected from her body and Mother Earth. Her human body did not feel right even though she woke up in it each day. While she was talking, I was guided to ask her questions.

The first question I asked was: "Did you have something happen when you were 4 years old?"

Her answer was "No." Then a bit later she said, "I think it was before my 5th birthday."

The second question I asked was: "What do you remember before you were 5?"

She said "Nothing." She explained that when she looked at family pictures, those taken before that age did not seem familiar. Then we went to the healing room.

What I needed to keep in mind was that I had not been trained in this area, but I was being shown something new. I had learnt to work with my spirit guide and follow directions. We did a session for her and provided for the first time a light body integration. After this, I was brought 2 more clients that were going through the same thing. They did not remember any of their life here before the age of a huge trauma. So I got more practice in and was shown how we can create a healthier vessel to live in.

Before our soul / spirit comes back to the Earth into a human body, we choose the family and life that we believe will help further us in our growth as a human being. With the human experience, the lessons can be very tough and long, until we understand and master what we need to learn.

There are times when one soul starts life in the human form, but due to the intensity of the lessons and situation the soul wants to leave. If it is for the highest good that this person stays here, then another soul will take that challenge to complete the life cycle of the human.

After the second soul enters the physical body, the person can feel like that new soul/spirit never felt comfortable in the body that it is helping out with. They feel detached. They wonder why they are here, and many times do not remember the life of the human before they entered to take over. Memories are very foggy.

Here is an example:

For the client mentioned above when she was almost 5 years old, there was a traumatic experience that happened in her family. This experience scared her so much that she wanted to leave. She did not want to experience this ever again. She was done with being a human, as such events were too harsh and damaging to her spirit and soul. She did not like the pain it caused, so her spirit left the physical body.

Now, this family needed this little girl. They needed her to be there so that they could carry on and finish their life mission, and the first soul had originally taken on this mission for that family. In that moment of the tragedy, another soul stepped in to take over the task of the first one. The second soul had no memory of the first 4 to 5 years. Even looking at baby pictures or pictures up to that age did not register. All the other pictures did after the 5th birthday. Something still did not feel right for her.

When we were in the healing room and this lady was lying on the table I got to see a soul line for the first time. Also I felt the imprints that were left behind by the tragedy, as the imprints were still in the physical form. This fully explained why this second soul did not feel comfortable, why it never felt it belonged in the body and the family seemed foreign. There was a lot of work to do for this person. Healing was required for the physical, emotional and spiritual. By the end of the session, this client felt a lot lighter. It still took another day or 2 for her body to adjust fully to all the energy changes and the new shift in her vibration.

After the session I explained everything that I saw and felt while the client was shifting on the table. After sharing with her that I had a strong feeling that she was the only one in the family that made healthier choices in life, it put all the pieces together for her. They needed her support to get through all that went on during that family's life. She was a gift to them. The first soul was to be there for this, but the task was too hard, and the second soul was strong enough to face the trials and traumas that followed.

This led to 2 other healings for walk-ins within a 2-month period. The universe wanted to make sure I fully understood what was going on and for me to see the different situations that souls are faced with while being here on Earth.

Present life with walk in of 2nd soul:

The bottom part of the body appears to be thick and heavy.

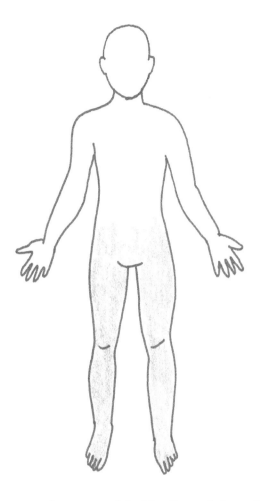

As the energy work was completed for the walk-in soul, the body felt more connected to Mother Earth and the heavens at the same time. The bottom part of the body was cleared, imprints healed and traumas released. Then we were guided to do the light body integration.

Chapter 6
....

Light Body Integrations and
DNA Adjustments

WHEN THE FIRST CLIENT CAME FOR HER WALK-IN ENERGY adjustment, a light body integration was also introduced to the training that I was receiving from my spirit guide and other beings of the universe. I am sure my Arcturian friends were very present in the room. I was getting a high five for listening and following directions. Training is needed for all of this as human-kind is starting to open up to further enlightenment, and best of all, natural healers are now more accepted in the western world. The western world has been so suppressed for too long and we are crying for change.

Again, with the light body integration, I found that the process helps the newer soul/spirit energy fit into the body better. This creates more of a glove-like feeling. When the integration is completed, the rest of the energy session is used to help release the past trauma in order for the client to finish this life time a lot more comfortably. Sometimes the integration will heal deep traumas that we could not pick up on at the beginning of the session.

The light body is the energy of the spirit. When the spirit is very strong, the energy feels really good. The energy extends throughout the whole body and beyond it.

Picture of healthy light body

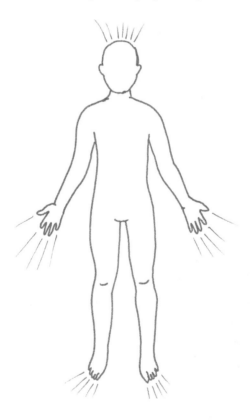

Many times during treatments for clients, you can get the sense that the person does not want to be here on planet Earth. The practitioner needs to do some clearing of the body first and make sure there are no entities or other heavier energies attached. This is done by bringing up the energy of the client and doing some cord cutting along with the safe removal of the heavier energies before proceeding. I have just gotten a strong feeling that the practitioner needs to have her/his own vibration quite high before attempting any of this and fully working from the heart centre.

The light body appears to be strands of light, like filaments. This light /spirit energy is very strong and very bright. It appears like strands of pure white light. This can also be defined as that spark we are of God/Creator energy.

This energy is first brought in through the crown of the client into their chest area. Once this has settled, the light filaments are brought into each of the arms, into the torso, then through each of the legs. During this process, the energy/light is so strong that the practitioner can pick up on other deep healing and or releases that are going on. The practitioner is guided when to go on to the next area.

At the end of the light body integration, the filaments extend beyond the finger tips, the toes and the crown (the top of the head.) The light body is big and needs to fit better into and beyond the human vessel. The body feels better, like it is wearing a customized body glove. When our vibration is higher, we feel a lot more comfortable, and there is less chance of any sickness settling in the human vessel. Remember: We are spiritual beings having a human experience.

I was just guided to add the DNA adjustments to this section. When we agree to live here, the vibration is different from our home planet or region of the galaxy. Due to life styles, trauma, blood contamination, and diseases, the human soul will have fragments of its DNA change over life times. I was just shown in a vision, that in the different regions of the galaxy the DNA can be different for the type of body and physical environment.

The physical environment can be the air, water and food available for us to live in. The DNA will accommodate the life-style and needs of the being for in the region that he/she is living in. An example would be if a person has a darker type of skin, the body will not burn so much in a hotter country. The fair skin person would be able to live in an area that had more rain with lots of cloud cover and cooler climate.

Another example of this was a person that I just worked with in March 2015. This person is a strong soul, been like a mentor/student/friend for a few years. He was going through a tough time, and I asked what could be done for him on this planet so that he could go forward again to be the teacher he was, more freely. What I saw and heard was that when he came here, he did not finish integrating his energy fully. There was a shift that needed to be done energetically with his DNA. I saw the process happen in a vision during the adjustment. I knew that the person needed 72 hours to allow the process to engage fully. Something we need to keep in mind with this is that we need to keep our living area and quarters in a high vibration so that our bodies will be and stay healthy on all levels. If we don't, we can get sick again.

During sessions, there have been a few DNA adjustments for the clients. At first I was taken aback and asked my spirit guide "Is this safe? Is it for the highest good?" The answer was yes to both questions. When the shifts/adjustments happen, I see the process, and I hope I can share this in some of the diagrams. I see a chain of the clients DNA. The DNA appears to be like a ladder with rungs/steps. Sometimes the rungs are crooked, or not in sync, or a rung is missing, or it could just be tainted. The DNA is adjusted by the higher forces of the light to the right calibration for the human is this life time.

DNA with missing rungs (1), broken rungs (2), and DNA corrected (3).

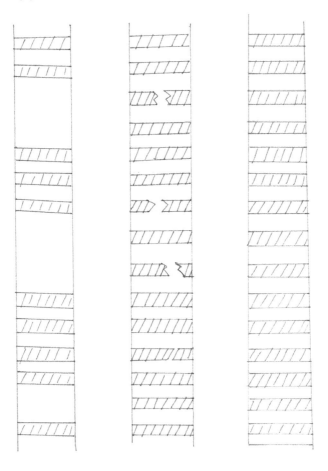

When I see the DNA adjust, it appears like a window blind shifting back and forth, until all the rungs are in the right place, properly spaced and fully repaired.

Once DNA adjustment is completed, the life becomes a lot easier health wise. This is one reason we must be very careful what we consume and put into our bodies. It is necessary to think about how we may be drinking alcohol, taking drugs, eating GMO food, and even using vaccinations? What are these things doing to our bodies? Is any of this changing our DNA? Are they toxic? We need to do things in moderation and look after our health on all levels.

Something to remember is that healing work for the body and soul with light body activations help the human body adjust better to the changing world around us. The vibration on planet Earth is getting higher due to us all working together to bring love and compassion back in to our world. Sometimes when we have just experienced a lot of learning or an influx of energy it does not sit well within, almost making one feel agitated and lost. The light body activation can help us integrate all the energies for our highest good. It also helps us go more into the heart centre of the divine love of source and reconnect again to the true essence of our souls.

Chapter 7

. . . .

The Truth About Spirits

NOW WE GET TO TALK MORE ABOUT SPIRITS.

I got quite excited when this chapter came up. When we get interested in numerology, synchronicity comes into play, and we see the significance of what we are doing. The significance of the number 7, is to learn about being able to trust and to be open to possibilities.

During the months of February and March, I kept seeing the number 3. When the body (physical), spirit and soul are balanced, we are in the state of divinity! I have been guided to place 3 dots on the animal friends in my batiks and drawings. My car accident landed on a 3 day, 3 bad dreams followed and led to this book. The sale sign for the house went up on a three day. This book was written on how we can heal the body, the spirit and the soul.

My birth number is 7. We are now in Chapter 7. The reason is to share the truth behind what I have learned over the years and to help others out. Following are some numerology explanations for when we are living a 7 path.

7. Open up to a point of faith in themselves and others: Trust and Openness.

7. Thought/consciousness.

7: Mental analysis, technicality, introspection, peace, poise, scientific research, spirituality, faith, trust, stoicism, refinement, wisdom, silence, "theories and fundamentals," feeling, deepening, mystery.

To find your birth number:

If you were born January 15, 1978, your birth number would be calculated as follows:

1 (month) + 1 + 5 (15 day of birth)+ 1 + 9 + 7 + 8 (the year of your birth) = 32. 3+2=5. Your birth number would be 5.

I was born in a 7 year and on a 7 day and it all added to a 7. 25/7 for me. There are three 7's in my birth numbers.

I just realized that accident I got into was on a three day.

The accident was on February 20 2015.

2 + 2 + 2 + 1 + 5 = 12 / 3.

I would also consider the three 7's in my birthdate to be significant.

7+7+7 = 21/3.

I would also consider the 3 outbursts I had with friends, the 3 bad dreams about entities and the 3 injuries that I got from the accident significant. Even though some of this may seem heavy, I see it as the end of one cycle and the beginning of a new cycle.

When I shared that I was going to record all of this, I got the following messages from 3 friends:

1. So cool Kimberley! Your 3's are also validation and encouragement for creativity and self-expression. You must sing your song and speak your truth.

2. Three is a very sacred number. I always have resonated with three. The mind, body and spirit. Trinity. The strongest shape is the triangle as it has 3 sides. All included in touching each side.

3. To be given the gift of consciousness. The infinite knowing.

Someone who is working with the number 7 is learning about trust and to be open, and a Pisces also learns to share the truth about what they intuitively see. A few years ago, after I developed my web site, I woke up one night remembering a profound dream. I dreamt about several people from all walks of life, working together to bring peace and harmony to the world. I was walking past a house, and saw 2 people talking. One of them looked at me and said to her friend, "Be careful of that one, she is a truth seeker, she knows.`` I was guided to place this name "Truth Seeker" on my website to learn the significance later.

As the years went on, I searched for the truth about the spirit realm and why the spirits showed up in so many different ways. I shared earlier that I was drawn to the spirit realm as a child, I had lived in fear of something that I did not understand. My recurring bad dreams caused havoc during the night and the energy of them sometimes continued into the day. During the dreams, it felt like I was being held down by something really strong. I could not move and always knew that something not nice was in the dream state. As a child, I could see spirits around my bed, this was not bad, but what I did not like was the energies that reached up from under the bed and beside the bed. These energies hurt me, poked me, and made me cry. I could feel the pain in the dream-like state. It was like lucid dreaming, I was aware, but I seemed to have no strength to fight back.

In 2005, I started to do clearings for houses to help shift the energy so that the houses would be more comfortable to live in. There were often energy imprints from abuse and sickness left behind. During these clearings, I would go into what I call Reiki mode, where I could pick up more about what was going on and do healing work for the rooms and furniture in the houses. Sometimes I knew if there was a female or male energy attached to the imprint and the cause of the discomfort left behind. There would be the odd cord cutting for spirits attached to the home.

In 2006, I started to have very bad experiences on the highway between Calgary and Cochrane. I would get very tired while driving down that stretch of road, for what seemed like no reason. It did not matter what time of the day it was or what the weather was like. I would bring food with me and something to drink, and I would even bite my fingers to stay awake. I started to get really scared. I knew I was not sick. I knew I was not crazy and I knew something was wrong. Then it happened. I almost fell asleep behind the wheel coming down a hill. I started to cry. When I got into town, I was heading for my home and was approaching a corner by the far end of the park where the kids did not normally play. I went out like a light in my car and then I hit the curb on the other side of the road. When I hit the curb, I came to. I was really scared. I could have hit a child. I got home, but I was terrified to get back into my car again.

It was the time to learn more about my dreams and why I was getting attacked in my car. Now 9 years later, I know that I am not the only one that this has happened to. That night I called 3 people. These people were aware of the spirit realm, and each one of them had an answer for me. This is what they shared:

1. Some of us are like a beacon for the spirit realm. Spirits come to us to help them cross over. We need to set boundaries as to when they can present themselves and as Manfred shared, we don't want to be one of them standing along the road in spirit form too. Later I learned more about Arcturus being a bridge to the other side.

2. The force that held me down is dream state, and the energy I felt in my car was spirit energy. It feels like a vacuum or a huge balloon pressing against you and sucks you into a dream/sleep state. It can feel like being paralyzed.

3. I needed to ask Archangel Michael to be with me on the highway. This was also during the time that I was learning more about the angel realm. I was to say when I got into the car "Archangel Michael above me, Archangel Michael below me, Archangel Michael in front of me, Archangel Michael behind me, thank you for your protection." From that day forward I have traveled with Michael and have been safe. I never again got that urge to have to take food and I know what to do when I get that sleepy feeling.

The next night I shared my experience with 2 friends that came by for a meditation. They suggested that the next time when I come back from the city, I should do Reiki while driving. This was only happening on the return trip.

On the way back a couple of days later I went into Reiki mode at the outskirts of the city and continued as I went down the road. With using Reiki it is the intention to provide healing for whatever may require it. About 200 feet or more east of Glendale Road (east of Cochrane), it felt like I drove into a vortex of energy. It was a weird feeling, but the energy felt familiar. As soon as I got to the intersection, I parked the car and got out. I asked for help so that I could understand what was going on. I did not see anything, but I could feel the energy of a whole bunch of spirits stuck there. A lot of them went right away, and some of them needed to do cord cutting. This process took about 5–10 minutes. When I felt that all the spirits had crossed over, my body relaxed, and then I said thank you for all the help and support. The rest of the drive home was a lot smoother. Over time, I heard that this intersection was really bad for accidents and deaths. I heard many stories and got lots of feedback. Since then I have never been bothered in that area.

From that time forward, when getting into the car, I always ask for protection. And at times when I felt that heavy energy, I would know right away to go into Reiki mode and pretend there was a huge sword coming from my car to do cord cutting.

There was only one other time that was as alarming, about 2 years ago. On the way to a work-shop that I was teaching in Lacombe, Alberta I had stopped at a set of lights at the first controlled intersection in town. Before I got there I was thinking of Archangel Michael. I wanted him to be with me. When the lights turned green I heard a car honk, and I was confused where I was for a moment, I realized that I had drifted off into a trance-like state. Shaken, I drove to Tim's for a coffee. I saw one of the students and asked if there had been a huge accident on the road in town. She said no. Later in the workshop, we were working with crystal energy, and I got a really strong feeling about something. I asked the students if something was going on in town in the direction that I was pointing to. They shared that there was work being done in the cemetery. That made sense! A spirit had come to me in the car to let me know they needed help. The next morning at home, I did a meditation and asked what I could do to help out. What I felt was that there were a lot of children that were buried there, knowingly or unknowingly and they wanted help going to heaven. During the meditation I did the cord cutting for the spirits.

Since 2006, I have been guided to help out a lot more with the spirit realm for the human spirits, and in 2011, the animal spirits started to ask for help too.

What needs to be shared is why spirits get stuck here. When we are raised with different religious beliefs, some are told that there is a heaven, and there is a hell. There is no such thing as a hell, as far as I am concerned. Many others will support this belief too. This place called hell was created to put fear in us. Fear that if we do wrong, if we don't succumb to rules, or specific thought patterns, or believed we were better than others, that we would not to go to heaven when we die. Many who have taught these beliefs were power hungry, or were so struck by fear itself, they led lives that they believed were perfect. They became very judgemental and created unhealthy thought patterns. Some were chauvinistic, some strongly disliked the opposite sex, and some discriminated against other nationalities and their beliefs.

When we are taught that we are going to hell, when the physical body dies, the spirit will stay in the area that it passed away in. The spirit stays stuck on the Earth plane. The spirit does not feel worthy of God's love and believes it will not get another chance. The spirit might stay on the side of a road, in a hospital, or in a house that it lived in. Sometimes the spirit might also be in denial of its physical body's death.

This is when I found that I needed to be in the heart centre, to truly show the same love and compassion that God would. I did not need to be scared of the spirits. An assistance and understanding were what was needed. Usually when I get a call, a family is being affected by what I will call the antics of a spirit.

The spirit is causing chaos by showing itself. Or sometimes the family members will start to feel angry, scared or even start to experience anxiety. The energy in the home has been disrupted. If left unresolved, the energy can cause divorces, sickness and more.

Imagine being in a space where no one can see you or hear you. You are alone, but you feel that you are not deserving of God's love or allowed in heaven. Then all of a sudden there is a couple or family in the physical space around you. There is the feeling of love. There is laughter, hugging, companionship, children running around, meals, family gatherings, and you can't partici-pate in any of it. No one can see you. You are being ignored.

When a spirit or a person feels this, the sense of being alone starts to sink in. Whether it is a spirit or human, the feeling of abandonment turns to resentment and anger. hen the spirit might start to lash out and cause chaos in the surroundings that it is in. The spirit still does not realize that it can cross over to the other side. That is when I get a phone call from those in the area that know what I do. When I go to the home where the spirit is stuck, we begin with a regular house clearing. When there is a spirit, my shoulders start to get sore. I can feel the energy along the top of my back, from shoulder to shoulder. As this happens, I know that it is time for a quick chat. When we can share with the spirit that God is waiting for him/her, and we can bring the love and light into the spirits energy field, then the spirit will let go. Sometimes Archangel Michael still needs to help cut the ener-getic cord of the spirit that is holding it back. Once the energy has fully shifted for the good, my shoulders relax and the energy feels calmer. Archangel Michael and his team assist in taking spirits to the other side, as soon at the spirit knows it is free to go to heaven.

Once the spirit has crossed over to the other side, the energy in the home or area will change, and it will feel a lot more peaceful. The little ones, the children, are more open to the spirit energy and usually will be the first ones to feel them and hear them. I have even watched them shift as a spirit leaves their home.

Sometimes spirits also get stuck here due to family members or spouses holding them back. When people pass away, it does not matter whether they are very sick or healthy, they can get stuck here, even when they know they can go to heaven. What can occur is that the people that are in deep mourning will not let the dying or dead person's spirit go. They hang on so tight that their health also goes downhill as the spirit energy can feel really heavy. This is hard on both the person that passed and the one that will not let them go.

I have just been guided to take this a step further, but this will be another chapter of learning.

Chapter 8
· · · · · · · · · · · · · · · · · · · ·

Spirits and Energies Who Became Lost

SOME SPIRITS CAN BE LABELED AS BEING EVIL, DARK, OR ALSO known as entities. These energy forms are unseen by most humans, but their presence can be felt by many without us knowing. This kind of energy again is created by unhealthy thinking patterns and actions. Again, when working with lost spirits and energies I needed to learn to be in the heart centre, but I had to take the healing a step further.

What has happened, in my belief, is that due to a spirit's evolution here on Earth, a spirit that has made many wrong choices will get darker with time. The choice could have been from abusing other people: life after life (or even in one specific life time.) Other choices could be have been from: participating in dark practices, or harming people or animals, or it created unnecessary chaos that took the lives of others. They could be the ring leaders who convinced others that they had the right to gain power through war or massacres. Those that participated or got brain washed, would not have the same energy but would still have to deal with the harm that they participated in later on, like a karma effect.

There are also what I see as entities and dark energies that come in different forms. Over the last 2–3 years I have been shown dark spirits, entities, demon-like energy and even had a demon spirit dog enter my home. You would wonder how such energy could come into a place where the vibration is so high, but it was something for me to learn from. When such energy comes into my home, it knows it is ready to make changes, to evolve to a higher vibration. It is almost like it is looking for redemption. The dark energy came in attached to a person that briefly stayed here. That person, I found out later, was heavily involved with drugs.

In 2014 when a client arrived, there was a dark spirit attached to her. A few months later another client came over for severe depression. Each experience was a blessing for us all: this was to learn how we can recognize what can enter our space, and both clients are now doing the same work I do.

Lost Spirits

The first client with a lost spirit had just come over for a visit. She had been feeling out of sorts for about 2 weeks, and she was feeling angry. When I had her stand up and started to smudge her, I could not stand still. My body felt like it was bouncing around her. We then went to the healing room and had her lie on the table. Starting with bringing in the Reiki energy, I started to ask her questions when I got to her heart area. Started her energy clearing and I got a really weird feeling. I asked where she was 2 weeks previous to that date, but I was not hearing quite what I thought was right. She said she was in the city, but that did not ring a bell, so I asked about here in town. Was there somewhere in town where she started to feel angry and did not want to stay in the building that she was in. Then it all clicked for her. She was at a store that carried both new and old products. She remembered talking to the owner and then getting into an argument before leaving. I went to the gal's right arm, placed my hand on her shoulder and the other hand on the lower arm. We needed to bring the light and higher vibrating healing energies, I also asking for Archangel Michael's help. When the process was done, I could feel the release of the spirit. During the process I knew this was a dark spirit, one that had been sent into a purgatory-like state because of its life choices.

About 5 minutes later I was drawn to look at the energy of the spirit that we just released, and he said "What the heck, I am with an Angel after what I did."

I said to him calmly, "You have a choice, what do you choose to do next? This is up to you." Then both the darker spirit and Archangel Michael left.

When Archangel Michael escorts spirits and entities out, he takes them to the next step. Some may go straight to heaven, some are safely disposed of or transmuted by white light, and others for further processing or review to see what had happened in that life time. Again, I believe that as a soul, all have many life times to learn and grow.

Dark energies and entities

Entities are created by unhealthy living environments, negative thinking, excessive drugs and alcohol. These things I generally see on the bottom of a person's leg. Finally after over 40 years of spirit dreams, I have realized that is what was hurting me in the dream state. When spirits cross over, the entities stay here as their energy is too heavy and unhealthy. With this new information, I am learning how to infuse them with light-healing energy to dissolve them, or if they are really big, I ask for assistance.

During a Reiki class that I was instructing, a student and I saw a big entity on the back of his friend. The entity, called an Arcon, it was in its' glory. It was getting stronger as it was sucking up the heavy energy that was being released from the others students during the Reiki practice. But it was also draining the person it was attached to. I tried at first to get it to leave, and then I stood in a stance and forcefully brought in the white light. I needed to make that stand, be strong and say to the Arcon, "This is not right. You are not allowed to continue to do this." When the vibration had changed, I asked for assistance again, and the entity was escorted out. After this, the student found that his back did not hurt anymore and that his intuition got stronger. At the end of the work-shop I asked the 2 students to stay a bit longer after the workshop, explained what I saw, what was done and how they could avoid having this happen again.

Another student came to the crystal healing workshop that I teach. Both of the ladies that attended worked as counsellors in a drug rehabilitation centre. We worked with about 50 different crystals over the day in the workshop. By the 4th crystal, one of the students was feeling queasy. She asked if we were almost done. We stopped and made her a peppermint tea to help sooth her stomach. I removed some of the crystals from the table wondering if the energy was too strong for her. When we started to work on the 5th crystal, I scanned her body and saw the entity on her leg. I infused the entity with white light and made sure there was no imprint left afterwards. When we shared what we felt with the 5th crystal, I did not say anything at the time, and she shared that she felt a lot more peaceful. At the end of the workshop, we discussed what happens in work areas and I provided some energy clearing methods for them to use with the crystals.

I have seen it in 2 people and had the demon dog in my home. This spirit dog was created from drug use that a tenant was involved in. He told me on the first day that he smoked cannabis, but he assured me that he would not do it around my home. The first week that he was here, when I came into my house from the side door, I looked down the stairs and saw for the first time a demon dog. The spirit dog had red eyes, and was smaller than the size of a husky, but it was still a big dog. I was shocked, and said to the demon dog, "I am sorry sweet-heart, but you do not belong here." I asked Archangel Michael to escort him out. Then I proceeded to do a full clearing of my home with sage and sweet-grass. When the fellow got home, we had a talk about what I saw, what I did and how to avoid such things. I did not want to bluntly accuse him of anything, but I wanted him to be more aware. At the end of the month I had to kick him out. I found out he was involved in heavy drugs, and this was not acceptable in my home or anywhere else. The use of drugs like that and excessive use of alcohol can both create bad heavy energies that affect people just as much or more than the substance used. A friend came over to ensure this person left, and we changed the locks. Again, a full smudging was done for my home.

This same demon-like energy, the red eyes, I have seen in the eyes of 2 different people. This kind of dark energy can create an electrical-like feeling when it is around. It feels heavy, intimidating, and makes you feel like you are sick to your stomach. You get a feeling like you don't want the person around, even though they are your best friend. What we were able to do with the first one was work as a team to bring in the light, change the vibration of the dark energy and ask Archangel Michael to escort him out and tell it not to return. What I mean by that, is when something is that dark, the chance of it turning back to light is slim. Those spirits / energies need to be 100% changed or sent to purgatory. No return. That way they can never harm or take over someone's space again. This was the same for the other person that I saw it in. The heavy energy needed to be safely changed and escorted out.

Sometimes we just don't realize what we are doing when we dabble in energies that we don't understand. These spirits can cause dark, heavy feelings for those who they come in contact with. These energies can try to control our thoughts and energy. They can bring thoughts of destruction and convince a person to do things that are not right. This brings me to another client and her so called friend.

A few months ago, I had a client come over for a Reiki session. She was depressed and did not know what to do. During the treatment, something felt off, but with the energy work she was able to release a lot of the sadness and other blocks that she had been holding onto. I shared what a beautiful soul she was and how I knew she was going to get her strength back. When we sat for a bit afterwards and chatted she had a very distant look in her eyes. This had me a bit confused as usually clients are radiating after a treatment and their eyes shine. As she went to her car, another friend of mine came in. While we were chatting, we both heard a huge bang outside and ran to the window. I knew something was so very wrong and I ran outside. I had this awful feeling about something else being in her vehicle but dismissed it. I did not want to think that it was unsafe for someone to come into my home. The client had crashed her vehicle into a lamp post after hitting a truck that was parked in front of her twice. I was crying and ran to her van. I looked at her. She was so dazed. I told her to turn off the car and get out of the van. I was scared of a fire starting. She had no idea what had happened. She said that it felt like she could not remember how to drive.

About a week later I called her, still scared for her. During our conversation, I shared what I felt when I ran outside and thought I was nuts. I also shared how I thought her vibration had gotten so much stronger that maybe a spirit did not like it. I had the sense that the spirit had stayed in her vehicle when she came into my house. She told me that a spirit had started to visit her years ago and would tell her to do weird things. It would get mad when she did not listen. It was mad she came here and it did stay in the van. I let her know that she needed to send it with the angels, that what the spirit was doing with her was wrong. She shared that the spirit felt that it was like going with the police if it went to the angels. We chatted for a bit more and I helped her to understand that this energy was creating the depression, and the spirit was trying to control her life. This energy was not there for her highest good and what it was doing was wrong. After doing some energy work for her over the phone, we were able to safely escort the spirit out. A week later she left an awesome message saying thank you for all the help and was so grateful that I had called. Now she is on the path, learning how to do healing work for both herself and others.

With these experiences, I started to understand more what was going on with the spirits and entities. When a spirit is ready to go, it will show itself on a client when they come for a healing session or the spirit will pass through at night (around 1:00 a.m.) when I am in dream state. When a spirit is stuck on a client, it helps to provide an opportunity for both the client and the spirit to heal. Sometimes it is just the matter of the client knowing that they are still loved and being looked after but from the other side. For the clients that pick up the dark spirits, it is a matter of bringing awareness of the places that the person goes into.

When the first friend came over, I had a feeling that her attached spirit knew that it had found a way out and knew my friend would come here.

From working with the spirit realm over the years and learning more about the entities, I have been able to put the puzzle together. The car accident that I was in helped me to understand that we can work to help spirits change and make healthier choices in their next life, but working with entities was a bit more intensive. After the accident that happened on a 3 day, I proceeded to have 3 dreams with entity energy in them. I realized that it was not the spirits bothering me, it was the entities being left behind. My energy is strong enough for the stuck spirits to go through, but the entities have not shifted enough and stay behind and scare the day lights out of me. The last time I had a dream where I sensed they were there I brought in the light to change their vibration. I did not get up angry and terrified about being hurt.

Learning to work with spirits and entities is very similar to working with a human or animal that has been scared or living a life that has been very hard. People who are raised in fear of survival, scared of where the next meal will come from, when the next beating or rape will happen, or when they will be yelled at or left behind, the person will grow up in a world of illusion or fears. They will create only what he or she believes that it deserves, or will harm others so that they feel the same pain. That is all the spirit or entity remembers. Even this energy can be healed.

Chapter 9

· · · · · · · · · · · · · · · · ·

Clearing of Energies

AGAIN, MY SPIRIT GUIDANCE IS TAKING DIRECTION WITH THIS book, and I fully understand why this information needs to be shared.

In Chapter 7, I mentioned how I needed to learn to be safe no matter where I went. We need to remember that when safe spaces are created, we become healthier and life gets easier for us and everyone around us. The energy becomes more divine and loving. When my car goes on the road, I ask for Archangel Michael's help so that the roads and area will be cleared for miles all around me, this is so that we are all safe. There are times when the Reiki and light energy is brought in, cord cutting for spirits is performed and still you must at all times use caution and be 100% alert.

When we think of the roads and highways, just think of all the accidents and mishaps that occur along them. People get angry, people drink and drive causing car crashes, injuries and so much more. Even when we pass some towns or cities, the energy is really heavy. Are we affected by this energy? Yes!

Several years ago, my oldest daughter and I were coming home along a country road. As soon as my daughter saw a small town, she shivered and said we had to keep going. The same feeling happened one time just west of Drumheller, Alberta. The feeling was awful. Right away, I started to do Reiki for the area, and about 5 minutes later, I felt fine. These all are energy imprints and entities. When the energy gets that heavy, we get a sick feeling in the belly. We get scared to stop, as fear had been created in that area. There are areas in Calgary, Alberta, were I don't like going. As soon as the car is there, or I get out of my car, I can feel the heaviness. These parts of the city have the highest crime rate, accidents and more reported deaths on the news.

I am sure that we can go to many cities and towns, and feel this kind of heavy energy. These areas are more in the industrial areas, gang-run neighbourhoods, and where there are a lot of bars and pubs. This is where people feel that they have come to the end of the road and can't see a way out of the lifestyle that they have.

Many times I have even walked into healing centres, hospitals, and home-based clinics where the heavy energy was so thick that it felt like walking in sticky tar. The first time I remember experiencing this was in a clinic in Airdrie, Alberta a few years ago. One of the rooms was the office of a therapist that worked with both children and adults.

What happens in areas like these, is that when someone is seeking help for physical, emotional and mental abuse, as they share or release the emotions that are tied to the event, they are shedding. Physical pain, emotional pain and mental pain hurts within us and can create discomfort on the outside of us too. These pains can cause discomforts such as breathing difficulties, rashes, sore joints and more. When we realize we can let it go, the pain sheds and goes to the floor. The energies of the heavens and angels are light, high vibration. Human energies that are from pain or sorrow are heavy, low vibration. Just think of it like gravity. The human body is weighted to the Earth. We can jump, but our weight brings us down again. This is the same as the pain energy that is released from the body. This energy falls and goes towards the floor. Then the mind and physical wellbeing feels lighter. We feel freer and like we are floating as if in meditation.

Now we are left with a pile of thick, sticky tar-like glue in energy form on the ground. When this is not cleared properly by light energy or sage, an imprint is left behind. After a bit, you wonder how patients were even able to heal in such conditions, or maybe the energy felt no different from what they were already feeling. Yet they always knew they needed to go back for more help. This can happen anywhere, but this is more common in centres that provide health care.

This is when I get a phone call and hear friends say "We needed help from the top guns." Now that I think of it, the top guns are the sage, energy work and the awesome angels that travel with me. We work as a team to help clear this energy safely and bring the light back in. When I work from room to room, I cannot physically leave that room until all the energy has been changed and all the imprints have been fully healed. When this shift occurs, my shoulders relax and I can move again. My body feels lighter. After the sage is used, then the sweet grass is lit and taken from room to room, and blessings are brought in.

For the times that I am going to another location to do workshops, I ask for help from the angels to provide a full clearing before getting there, and I can also send light energy to the area. That brings up the energy, and this provides a more peaceful energy there. In my home, I do a lot of clearing after clients and smudge if furniture gets moved around or if someone comes by and leaves a sadness or anger behind.

The same can be applied to houses and other buildings. Even the furniture and fixtures in these places can carry energy. I have been in homes where there are weird locks on basement doors where I could feel that someone was locked in down there. The energy in these spaces can bring goose-bumps to your arms and an overwhelming sense of sadness. I have worked with furniture that held the anger of the previous owner. There was a bed that someone died in, and a couch that a sick person had lain on during a lengthy illness. I believe we had a second hand chair in our office that had a spirit attached to it, as each time I sat in it, I fell asleep and had a hard time waking up. One house had a brass coat rack, and even though it was beautiful, it felt awful. I visited a home that had imprints from physical abuse on the bedroom and was told later that there was a huge blood stain in the carpet when the new owner bought the house. When I walked into that room, I got goosebumps and felt scared, like I had to keep looking over my shoulder.

Over time, abuse can leave impressions behind, even though the people have moved out. You can feel these entities, the emotional imprints: it all feels horrid and can have an effect on the next occupants. Happy, loving couples and families can move into places like this, and then they proceed to get angry, sick or even get a divorce without knowing why. Always try to check into the history of your new home or business before moving in.

I would highly recommend that any property be smudged before taking residence, even if it is a new home or office building. Sometimes land is not obtained with integrity, previous owners don't want to move on, or there may have been deaths from long ago battles. We need to help heal the land and anything that is on it.

During a house or business clearing the owners are with me as we go from room to room. They will stay in the hallway while I work but they will notice where I get stuck and spend a longer time. After each clearing I share what I picked up on, and then they share that I got stopped at the same spots they had trouble with. Each clearing brings in much better energy and the lives of the families will be smoother and they will be a lot happier. As I do the clearings, I share what I do with the sage so that the owners can be aware of what they can do themselves if smudging is required at a later date.

We especially need to be aware of what we bring into our homes. Clothing, furniture, old toys, books and old tools can all carry a heavy energy with them. Pictures that hung on someone's wall during war time or from a home with severe depression or anger can affect your home with their sadness. Many times, people don't realize what is going on until weird things start to happen in the object's new home. A person could be loving and kind, until they put on the sweater that they got at the garage sale. Or enter the room with the used toys, and start getting sad or angry. This is how quickly something can change our feelings and well-being.

About three years ago, I needed to share my bedroom with a family member for a few months. Not long after the young one had moved her bed into my room, I started to get really bad dreams. These dreams were not the spirit dreams: they were dreams that I could not remember and would wake the young lady up too. Four months later, while listening to a conversation, I realized what was going on. I was picking up on the young lady's dreams. When asking her if she had a lot of bad dreams, she started to cry. This could be why she never wants to have her own bedroom. A few crystals, amethyst, selenite, kyanite and soda-lite were placed on a mat and then put under her bed. The bad dreams that I was picking up from her stopped. About a month after that I realized that when I went into my room at night, all I could feel was resentment. The resentment was created by the little one because I required that the room stay tidy. Needless to say, both the granddaughters were moved into my room, and I moved into a smaller room for the duration of their stay. They were then both comfortable, and I slept a lot better.

The energy of people and animals can easily transfer to things around us. This energy can affect solid objects, houses, land, vehicles and more. We need to pay attention to how we create our space. When we bring in love and light, the energy is loving and healthy. When we are not happy, hurting others or ourselves, the energy can be very unhealthy and harm others. Each time I go for a walk, I like to bring in and imagine that God/Creator light is coming in through my crown from the heavens, travel-ling through my body and down to Mother Earth. As I walk down the sidewalk, a path of love and light is being created along my journey. We can all do this! As we walk, go in a boat, in the car, even on a plane!

Chapter 10

Healing for Humans and Animals

I AM GOING TO SHARE MORE ABOUT WHO WE ARE AND WHAT we are capable of as both humans and animals. This journey of healing has become my heart song. This is something that has been on my mind for many years, and it is where I travel to each day. I am always asking God / Creator, my spirit guide and the angels what we can do to help out mankind, the animal kingdom and mother earth.

Each and every one of us is capable of providing healing energies for ourselves and others. When we share a hug, when we send a blessing, when we smile, sing or laugh, it is all a form of energy healing. Each one of us has a spark of God energy within us. Each one of us can create amazing, beautiful changes and bring in the love and light, when we are ready to be that love and light. Many have brought beautiful music, art-work, and dance to the world. When we engage in the arts and this energy, our hearts are uplifted, our souls sing and we vibrate in a healthy environment and body. We can also access this in silence, in a room or outside when we are alone. Peacefulness can bring a stillness to the mind.

As I write this information down, my belly gurgles energy. My higher self is happy that I am sharing. I feel good, happy and content. My tummy does the same when energy work is being done on me or when I work with clients. The rumbling sound can get really loud, yet the tummy feels happy, like my heart centre. As mentioned much earlier in the book, I was first introduced to a natural healer around 1997. As she was learning new healing techniques, I happily volunteered, still not quite sure what was really going on, but I knew this energy stuff to be helpful. The energy healing was helping me out and getting me through some tough times. I also knew that I needed to eat better, and start taking some additional B vitamins.

Human Healing

There are many forms of energy healing that have been or are taught around the world now. Energy work was been used in the Native cultures and the Eastern cultures for thousands of years. However, for many years, in some European countries, and during the early years of Canada and the United States, natural healing was frowned upon. Fear was placed into society stating that only the heads of the religious organizations that had a direct link to brother Jesus and God could do healing work. People who did not go to school like the doctors, but were interested in herbs had insights into the truth of what is, or used methods of energy healing, were judged and called witches. Many natural healers were burnt at the stake, hanged, drowned, and even their homes were burnt. Many of these amazing people were natural healers like the Shaman or medicine women of the Native culture.

Now in both countries we have access to many methods of holistic and natural healing practices. Some of these practices are Reiki, Therapeutic Touch, Healing Touch, Craniosacral Therapy, Acupuncture, Acupressure, Reflexology and even Counseling. Reiki was developed by Dr. Usui in Japan and then brought over to America and taught here by Mrs. Hawayo Takata. Acupuncture and Acupressure are from the Asian culture using the meridians of the body to release blocks to help heal the organs. Craniosacral Therapy was developed by Dr. John Upledger in the U.S.A. Therapeutic Touch was developed by nurses: Dolores Krieger and Dora Kunz. Now the American countries have many healing methods available to them, but there is still a lot of fear that people are holding onto.

There are many other forms of healing, but to list all of them is another book in itself. I will use the Reiki as a starting point. When I first started actively and knowingly learning about the different healing methods I started with Brain Gym. I saw some really neat changes, but it did not feel like it was my way of working. I needed to remember things like a doctor. Then I was introduced to meditative healing, and that one felt a little more comfortable: I could just be me. I did not need to follow any sort of instructions: it was just a knowing. Next was the Usui Reiki system of healing: this was what got my heart singing loud. I took the first 2 levels with an instructor, left with little paper-work and did both workshops in an afternoon. This was a stepping stone and a lesson for later when I was qualified to start instructing the workshops. The next Reiki Master that I learnt from really opened my eyes, answered a lot of questions and showed me how to incorporate some Native practices into the healing work. She also taught me the true value of a Reiki hug. This hug was unconditional love and healing energy all at once and started to open my heart again.

When we use energy, what I call Reiki energy, God/Creator energy we are bringing this healing in as unconditional love and healing light. Nothing on this planet is stronger than pure unconditional love and light. The vibration of this energy is so high and strong that it can and will change the heavy energies back to their original state. Let's use a bruised apple as an example. The apple got bruised because it was harmed by an external force. The rest of the apple is okay, but that one area has lost its vibrant taste and is soft, sort of lifeless. This can apply to the human body, when one bangs a toe on a table leg (I did this a few times about 10 years ago to get the lesson), your toe will bruise, swell and change colors. Greens, yellows, and purples show up in the bruise. It is amazing how colorful the body can be. But when healing energy is applied to the area right away, there is less bruising and swelling as the energy keeps the blood flowing, and helps to release the discomfort. Just like a team that is put together for trauma victims, they are there to provide support and show that the person is protected and being looked after. In both cases, the body is able to shift the energy and heal much farther. Like with the little toe, when Reiki is applied right away, the healing process is much faster.

Reiki and other forms of energy work can help to heal the body faster, but also help the body heal from past traumas. When we use the energy and tap into the soul/heart state of the human body, the energy will go to the areas that are seeking help. When someone is on the healing table, it is the client that is doing 90% of the work, and the practitioner is the vessel for the energy to flow through. This energy has a mind of its own. Unconditionally, it will seek out where the blockages are and help to release them and heal the body. This energy has no sense of judgment. It is the pure love/life energy from which we were created. The energy likes to be able to flow freely throughout the body, and if its journey is restricted, it will work on that area till it is freely flowing again. Many times people need to do healing sessions over a period of time, for their bodies to adjust to their new state of being. One layer is healed at a time.

When we are born, our third eye, or psychic ability is already pre-determined for that life time. As an example, the Arcturians are very telepathic and have a strong sense of knowing. As children grow up, they may have people around them that doubt what they see, hear and feel. After a while, the children will block out these senses so that they can be normal like everyone else. Or they may see things that scare them as a child and don't learn how they can work with these gifts or senses that they were born with. Each time something happens and it scares them, they may add another layer to block off the third eye. If I were to have had my third eye opened fully the first time that I was worked on energetically, I would have been scared out of my shorts. Then I would have gone back to that state of being closed off again. My mind and body needed to adjust to the changes, insights, visions, and the knowing that got stronger day by day. I needed to trust and learn to see differently and to know it was okay. This is what brought me to where I am today. Now when things are presented like dark energies, entities and all the scary stuff, I know that I am stronger and don't need to be scared. The opening of the third eye took a few years and I am still learning how to use the information I receive. This is like going through an apprenticeship.

Energy can help to heal injuries that occurred in the present time and the past. An injury from the past is like an imprint of the past event, and the body will hold onto that injury until the emotions are healed. An example of that is a reoccurring shoulder pain from the time the person was 12 years old. The child could have gotten hurt in a playground from a bully teasing and pushing other kids around. The person may have gotten better as a child, and the injury supposedly healed, but any time that person experiences anger from the actions of another person that does not show compassion, the shoulder can flare up again and cause pain. What needs to be done is to heal that imprint towards that anger from the original incident in the playground and provide forgiveness to the person that was being a bully.

Many times we hold onto anger and resentment, instead of forgiving the person for not acting in a more gentle way. What did that other person live with? What type of life style did that person have to experience? Was there abuse at home? When we go to our heart centre and learn to see others in a different light, and even ourselves, we start to see amazing people within the exterior shell that we created. Once that forgiveness is shared, verbally or in writing, that energy block can start to be released.

Over the last year I have been in 2 situations where my body was physically hurt. The first time was a dislocated shoulder, and the second time was a car accident that caused a concussion and fractured bone in my right hand. I want to go through the rest of my life without the discomfort of the accidents and want a peaceful state of mind. With the shoulder, there was a lesson on how others can misdirect their anger and the damage that can be done. I was the recipient of those anger spears that were thrown. Right before the anger spears were thrown, I was hoping the best for this person and someone else that had come to mind. Both of these people did not realize what they were creating around them with their actions and habits. When I got hit with the anger spears I was not paying attention to where I was walking and slipped in some melting snow, hit the ground hard and dislocated my shoulder. I knew right away what had happened and was shown by the angels that I was being looked after. I forgave and prayed for the best for the person that was angry and hoped that they would walk in the light again. I took very good care of my body and stayed in a good state of mind. About 8 months later, a good friend did some massage and energy work for me. She was amazed how well my arm had healed.

This will be the same for the car accident. To see the accident as an event that may or may not have needed to happen. To count my blessings that I was able to walk out of my car after it was hit head on and forced into the ditch. This accident was when I was driving full speed on the highway. I am so grateful that I am here today, and I am grateful for the other driver's sake that I made it out alive. I am very grateful, even though it was the other drivers fault, that my life was spared. If my life had been taken, that would have been a heavy load for that young driver to carry for the rest of her life. Also, I felt a lot of gratitude for paying attention and avoiding a much more serious accident.

When we can fully heal on all levels, physically, mentally, emotionally and spiritually, our bodies will thrive and be very healthy. I have learnt not to hold onto grudges and anger. I have always been very independent, very stubborn and rarely did I fit in with other people. I am more of a loner and I know that being around others can be hard, as I could feel the energy of what they were projecting and did not feel comfortable around bullies, those who discriminated against others and those who physically harm others.

I always tried to be soft-spoken and gentle. When my darker side, and my anger came out, I was embarrassed and ashamed of what I projected. Right away I would apologize. I do not like to hurt others, and I did not want them to feel awful for what I had done. We need to learn and know that we can't control others by harming them, physically, mentally, emotionally or spiritually as this all will cause an energy imprint or block that they will carry throughout their lives until they are able to recognize it.

Humans are also affected by mental abuse and words that are said by others because they don't want another to succeed or think they are better than the person they are attacking. Words such these: "You are stupid." "You don't know anything." "You are ugly." "You can't draw." "You can't do anything right." "No one else will like you." This kind of behavior is not acceptable, and many times, when we look at the person who is saying this kind of stuff, they were treated the same way as a child by another sibling or parent. The person that is being the bully, often has low self- esteem and wants to be looked at as better than others as they are not getting that support at home. Both my brother and I were physically and mentally abused for about 3 years, and I made sure that I did not repeat that pattern. We both were left with a lot to deal with and had to learn how to heal within. I provided my children with support, no matter what they were doing and let them know that I loved them, regardless of how they were acting. We need to learn to take responsibility for our own actions and to respect others. We need to think before we lash out towards someone else.

With this being shared, when we have turmoil going on in our bodies, and cannot remember why we walk in fear, why we feel ashamed of our bodies, or why we feel that we are not smart, we can learn to energetically release these patterns. When I have a client on the table for a Reiki session, we are connected soul to soul. The client's soul/higher self is able to guide me to an image or a knowing of where the harm occurred. Many times, we are able to recognize the age of the person or how many years ago the tragic event occurred. We can see an event or get a sense of what happened emotionally during this time. I ask questions that I am guided to ask. This helps the person to be part of the healing on a conscious level. The client's subconscious mind shows what needs to be healed. As the client answers the questions, the healing starts as the block or imprint is released. Sometimes, we need to do a soul retrieval for the client as the imprint is stronger, and we need to heal the fragmented parts of the soul for the person to become whole again. When we energetically heal the past, the present and the future will go a lot more peacefully. It will be easier to see ourselves as that perfect person that is a spark of God/Creator. Our bodies and mind get stronger.

Again, when we are doing energy work, we are bringing in the unconditional loving and healing energies of God/Creator, so that the vibration of the person on the table becomes stronger, and the heavy energies are changed back to light energies. When the client is on the table, they are doing 90% of the work. The practitioner is doing the rest by being the vessel for the energy to flow through. Practitioners need to be healthy, as the energy will heal us along with the person. The stronger the practitioner is, the more the recipient will receive. This healing energy is like electricity that flows as it is being channeled through. It is just like turning on a light switch. When the light switch is turned on, the light goes on. When the light switch is turned off, the light is out and there is no flow of energy. At the end of the session I make sure that the client is still connected to the source of light and not me.

Something to keep in mind: the human body has 7 major chakras. Many workshops go over the chakras and how they are related to our health. When our chakras are cleared and vibrating, our bodies will be healthier on all levels. When the chakras are blocked, our bodies get sick, and the different organs can be affected too.

Seven Chakras

Chakra one: The right to have **Root Chakra** (Pelvic area)

Survival, clothing, shelter, warmth, medical care, healthy environment, and physical touch are all a necessity of life.

Chakra two: The right to feel **Sacral Chakra** (Belly button area)

We all are individuals and are all sensitive in different ways, and we need to respect ourselves and each other for this.

Chakra three: The right to act **Solar Plexus Chakra** (Just below the ribs)

Our intuition tells us how to act in different situations. When we follow someone else, we may not be doing what is right for us. Our intuition is also a warning system for us to follow.

Chakra four: The right to love and be loved **Heart Chakra**

Hurt and rejection from parents, siblings, relatives, and others can affect our heart. Judgmental attitudes towards each other can also have an effect. We need to learn to love ourselves for who we truly are.

Chakra five: The right to speak and hear truth **Throat Chakra**

Unable to speak up and to defend ourselves, because we are scared of others reactions. When we speak from the heart, the words are kinder, and the message is stronger.

Chakra six: The right to see **Third Eye Chakra**

When we see things, or premonitions of events, we need honor that. We all have the ability to use our psychic abilities, yet many hide from fears.

Chakra seven: The right to know **Crown Chakra**

We have the right to education, knowledge and spirituality. We have our own beliefs, and we should not impose our beliefs on others.

Healing for the animals

Animals also are affected by abuse: physically and emotionally. I cannot speak for animals in their natural wilderness and how they are affected when they are harmed. In this situation it is more on the survival of the animal and if they are supported by their clan.

Animals that are taken by humans as pets, or as work animals, do show signs of abuse and over-use. The abuse can come from a bully human, from being raised in breeding mills or in feed lots, or from being used for races and championships. Animals are just like humans. When they are neglected and physically harmed, they too will lash out. Or some will become extremely timid and hide from anything that comes near them. They will hold onto the same lack of trust that a person can. Animals can also bring with them the hurt from the abuse from another owner.

Animals are amazing to work with energetically. They don't question what is going on with the energy and willingly receive the healing. When working with animals, practitioners can tap into the soul / heart line and help to release the imprints. They don't need to hear key-words, or know what is being energetically released; they love the calmness of the energy and will show signs of shifting. Horses will let out gas or even sneeze when they release old energy. Dogs and cats may just melt under the practitioners' hands and keep coming back till they feel they are done. Animals will even come to people for healing energy.

Once out at a friends' farm, where I had been doing a lot of weeding in the vegetable gardens, an owl was waiting on a hay bale for me. I was the only one that actively did energy work at the farm, and when I had arrived, I was told that an owl had been sitting on a hay bale by the gardens. Later when I went over to that section, the owl was still sitting there, in broad day light and with people around. This just does not happen. One of the workers cautioned me, but I knew I was okay. Right away I went into Reiki mode and sent energy to the owl. What I had sensed, was that the owl had hurt his wing. After awhile, the Reiki energy stopped, and I thanked the owl for being there. Later that afternoon he flew away. It was like the owl knew someone would be there for him that day.

Our dog, Romeo, was also a recipient of energy work. At first, the energy was too strong for him, so my hands were held above him. He always knew what I was up to and always stood still for me. When working with horses, we can stand away from them or do hands-on healing. There was an older work horse that I had to stand away from when doing energy work. He was a big horse that made friends with the female horse that came to the farm first. It took awhile, but he knew who he could trust and who would not hurt him. After a bit of the Reiki, Thor would come right up to me for pets and cuddles. We can help to release old fears and the imprints from the animals too so that they can lead healthier lives.

Chapter 11

The Other Realms

SO FAR WE HAVE DISCUSSED THE ANGELS, GOD/CREATOR, AND humans. Then there was a bit on the darker energies that have been created by unhealthy patterns or thinking. Both humans and animals have a solid physical body form. The angel realm and God are an energy form, but at the same time they have the essence of colour, thought, size, and form. These beings are energy forms that are of the in-between world. This is the spirit realm. And some would say this is only in our imaginations.

When we are young we are able to see the spirit realm better, until someone tells us that it does not exist because they do not believe in such things. My granddaughter saw both angels and fairies when she was little. My grandson saw a dragon-like energy in his kitchen when he was small. I have seen, as an adult, energy orbs, twinkles (sparkles of light), and client's spirit guide. I have felt powerful spirit animals in my back yard and the demon dog on my stairway. I have felt the hands of angels, heard my spirit guide give answers and more. Over the years having to relearn what I felt as a child, and I am learning even more now. I would love to see all the realms, but in the meantime, I can feel them or know when they are around.

Angels

The angels were the first to show themselves. With the instructor at the Angelic Awakening workshop, while she was talking about Archangel Raphael, I saw a green energy to the right of her with the shape of a head and shoulders. Another student saw the same thing. This was my introduction to the angel realm. I could feel the hands of the angels on my right shoulder when I was nervous driving in the snow in the winter time. Once when I came out of surgery, I wished someone was there with me, and I felt a big male hand hold mine. I was the only one in the room. Angels started to show up themselves with clients. I did not see them, but I could get a knowing vision of what they were wearing. Many times I shared with the clients what I was sensing around them. This was something they had heard before, or had seen themselves. We have guardian angels that are always with us, but they will never interfere in our journey. They will provide signs for us, but it is up to us to pay attention.

There are people that come for sessions that are what we call Earth angels. I can see their wings, and each set of wings is a bit different. Some are pure white, some have hues of brown like an owl, and some are almost bird-like. Angel wings are really thick with feathers, and massive. These Earth angels are here to help us in the transition from the dark ages back into the time of enlightenment. They are amazing humans with their hearts open and loving, and they are all very sensitive to what is going on around them.

I have worked with the angels for many years. Archangel Michael is like my brother. We work together as a team when we do house clearings, travel on the roads and any time I need extra strength to go that extra step. The first time I did a clearing for the entity I asked him to be at the house that I was going to, to encase the entity before I got there. After I had done the clearing, the ladies let me know they felt the angels come into the room shortly after they called me. Ten minutes later I was at their house with sage and sweet-grass, and the angels were already there to help do the clearing.

Archangel Raphael is another angel that I get to work with quite often. Archangel Raphael helps me with the cord cutting by sealing in the area where the cord was, helps me with the journey of becoming spiritual teacher, and with helps me when giving presentations on holistic work.

There are a few times when I have gone somewhere and asked that the angels be with me and I have felt them. Once, when going to see a medium, I asked for support while there, not knowing what a medium really did. Before the medium could get started, she told us that she had to adjust to the energy from the angels. At a couple of drum circles that I went to in Calgary, the lady leading the circles always said thank you to me at the end of the drumming for bringing in the angels. During one drum circle I could feel and knew that the elders in spirit form were in a circle outside the group of drummers, and the angels were in the outer circle.

The angels are here to help us out. They will never interfere in our lives, but they sure will provide some awesome messages when we are ready to receive them and go forward. We can ask them for help and support. We can work with them as a team till we feel we are strong enough to do things on our own. I know I had the angels with me many times. One time, while walking past a church during their service time, I started to talk to the angels and share that I knew that God was with me no matter where I went. All of a sudden, it felt like there was a huge team of angels beside me and behind me. The feeling was amazing, my back got straighter and I knew I was at the right place at that time, and knew I did not have to be sitting among the congregation to be with God. The angels are here to help us!

Fairies

Next I started to learn about the fairy realm. I was told many years ago that the fairies liked it in my back yard: they enjoyed the plants, the trees, the squirrels and birds. That was an honour to hear, yet I had never seen them. I have had friends bring fairy ornaments as gifts, and I just remembered the book that I bought on fairies when I was 18 (which my oldest daughter has now). When my granddaughter was little, she saw the fairies around my oldest daughter. My first known experience with the fairies was when the bottom of my legs got icy cold while working on a client. No doors or windows were open, and my legs were very cold. I asked the client after the treatment if she had fairy ornaments in her home. She did! She had several of them, and the message was that she was being supported by the fairy realm. During one Reiki workshop, I needed to gently ask the fairies to stand back and let their human friend have lots of space while learning. This was amazing to feel and know. Later this gal shared how she helped the bees out in the spring time by supplying water and sugar for them. The bees and fairies work very closely together.

The fairies are the keepers of the Earth plants and floral. They are here to help us too. They remind us to stand up for ourselves, to be true to ourselves and to learn to play again. I have sensed them among my plants in the house, outside in the gardens and out in Waiparous, in the forest. The ones that I sensed there were the tree climbers. On one visit there I got a glimpse of their movement in the lower bush and higher in the trees. My oldest daughter has pointed out their presence too. Their energy feels strong in the forest.

It is not often that a client comes over, that has strong fairy energy. Only two of them had fairy wings, and they were amazed, yet not surprised by the energy that I had sensed was with them. They are both grounded and pure of heart.

Animals

In 2010, at the end of the year, I went on a trip to Australia. When traveling around, it seemed that I was more connected to the animals than I had ever been before. This trip opened an amazing door for me energetically. In Sydney, a lorikeet (multi-coloured bird) kept landing on my leg, on the last day at my Aunty's house. While visiting a tourist centre in the Bunya Mountains, north-west of Brisbane, a wallaby really surprised me. While I was watching the wallaby (smaller than a kangaroo), it seemed like something weird was sticking out of it. At first I thought it was part of the male reproductive system. Then when I looked again, I said in a gentle voice, "Hey sweetheart, is that a baby in your pouch?." I was looking right at her. She slowly turned her body and showed me the little one that was peeking out. She looked very proud. I thanked her, and of course the relatives thought I was a little loony.

After the trip there, my dreams and the things that I was picking up on started to shift again. One night after I lay down, fully awake, I could hear something climb up the side of my bed. I was scared, but I so wanted to connect more with the spirit realm that I stayed really still. As I listened to the animal that was climbing up the side of the bed, it slowly walked along the top of my head. I realized that it was a kitten. The kitten sniffed my face and then it settled in for the night. By the time the kitten got settled I was out like a light. That is how spirit energy affects me. This led to other visits from the animal kingdom at night and the odd one during the day. One night I heard a big bear at the bottom of the bed, and a lynx settled in on my tummy. Two times a bird landed on my feet, his talons holding onto my toes. With all of this going on, I realized that the animal kingdom is here to work with me, but I also needed to help them out energetically. One night, a whole bunch of them came to the bedroom and then went running down the hallway to the living room. The next day, I did a lot of Reiki for them. I have never seen the spirit animals but I either know who they are, or I recognize who they are by their breathing patterns.

Each person has a totem animal that joins him or her at the time of birth. Once in a while, a person may have 2 totem animals, but that is rare. About 6 months ago, I was blessed to have a long visit with a Shaman. This Shaman was one of the three that let me know about spirit energy and helped me out. We chatted about animal totems and helpers, and how we needed to nourish our bodies properly, especially during a pregnancy. His theory was (and I fully believe him), that many pregnancies' don't come to term because the mother is not eating properly, or she is eating something that is making the unborn and developing child really sick. The mother is not eating what the animal totem requires for both her and the baby. This makes sense, when I was carrying my first child I could not be anywhere near meat, as the meat was not organic, and the smell was sickening, from what we now know to be the hormones and antibiotics in the meat. If the meat had been organic, my body would have reacted differently. My daughter also had skin sensitivities and could not be around any chemicals or perfumes.

Over the last few years, family members would bring me things that had a wolf on them or wolf ornaments, without knowing why. Once at the Body Soul & Spirit Expo in Calgary, a fellow vendor approached me and shared, "I am not sure where you are from, but I see you on a different planet, and you have a wolf with you. I have never seen this before." Of course I was honored to hear this. Even my granddaughter has gifted me with some awesome wolf ornaments and a wolf screen saver. When chatting with the Shaman, on the way to the TV show that a friend was doing with me on Spirituality, I mentioned a meditation where many animals came forward: the wolf, a deer, a cougar, a hawk, a raven and an owl. The neatest sensation was when they all shuffled around me to find a comfortable spot to be. Once we were all settled, it was like being a totem pole. I shared my theory that when we need help, or when we are making a shift in life, the spirit animals will join us to help out during the transition. He seemed comfortable with this thought. During the show, Manfred shared that I had both the Wolf and the Fox as totem animals.

I will share a bit about each of my totem animals, so that you have an idea of what I get to work with and how the information has helped over time.

Wolf

- The wolf is the teacher and also represents loyalty, guardianship and spirit.

- The wolf allows us to teach the medicines of the land for a healthier community.

- The wolf helps us to teach children the respect and lessons needed for growth and a humble existence.

- The wolf's loyalty brings us back to our home and origins.

- The wolf brings the people together for growth and lessons.

- The moon and the wolf are connected and both tap into the wisdom and psychic energies that we all can be a part of as we seek deeper wisdom.

- The wolf helps to bring back memories of the ancient ones.

- The wolf is not a fighter, but it will let you know when you have over stepped boundaries.

- When you work with this wise teacher, you learn that when you step into your shoes and truly embrace your gifts, you can be proud of who you are and you don't have to prove it to others.

- The wolf teaches us how to watch body language and to listen to the voice.

- The wolf's senses: smell, knowing and sight are very strong, and this can help to pick up on dangers and those who do not travel in the heart centre.

Fox

- The fox represents camouflage as the fox is able to blend into its natural environment. He is able to sit in the background and just observe while others are involved in their own activities.

- The fox also provides protection for the family unit. He / she is able to watch over the family and ensure that no one comes into danger.

- Fox medicine can teach us to observe, and watch, rather than get involved.

- The fox also teaches us how we can use many methods of healing: the animal kingdom, angels, God, crystals, and herbs. The fox is able to go into the other realms. The fox has the magic of connecting to the fairy realm, and supernatural power.

- The fox also represents femininity, and will show even the males that they need to be in touch with both their male and female energies.

Both the wolf and fox messages were affirmations of what I have been learning over the years. A lot of the messages can apply to many of us, yet have more of an impact when you know they are your totem animals.

The animal spirits and fairies seem to be more of Mothers Earths energy. They too are amazing teachers and helpers. Mother Earth's medicines help us to heal physically and emotionally. When we have a healthy combination of all the above along with healthy thought patterns we can be in balance physically, mentally, emotionally and spiritually. If you find that an animal keeps appearing, see what you can find on them, you just may have an awesome message coming your way.

Other spiritual helpers

During sessions with clients, we have many visitors, but many times it depends on who is on the table. We all work together for the highest good of the client. I will at no time take credit for doing the healing work: this work is a shared event and is always done for the highest good. Our visitors do help out and contribute with sharing their energies / essence and knowledge. I have felt the angels, fairies, elders, animal kingdom, sisters and brothers from neighbouring planets, the White Brotherhood (Brother Jesus is a part of this group) and what I know as the tall light beings. A friend mentioned that they were a silvery colour. Their energy is very strong. I don't always know who is sharing the information, but only those of the purest intentions and light are welcome.

About 3 years ago, I had a student that came for Reiki One and Reiki Two. During our first workshop when he tried to practice Reiki on me, he was energetically pushed away from my head. He commented and was a wee bit confused. The second time, he was pushed really hard and hit the closet door that was about 2 to 3 feet away from the healing table. This time, being mad, he said he couldn't work on me. Trying to figure out what was going on, I explained to him that we had many helpers in the healing room from the spirit realm and that we all are to work together. After this, we were able to continue the workshop. He success-fully worked on me. A few months later, we found out that there was another energy that was co-existing in his body other than his spirit and soul. We did a light body integration and escorted the energy out. This energy was not of the light and wanted to cause me harm during the workshop. That is why we needed to chat about the helpers and share that I was being protected in the healing room.

Some may still try to say that all of this is hocus pocus stuff, but after many experiences, clients and friends that have gone through all of this with me, know that there is much more to be seen. Things that fears have held us back from. When new learn-ing comes forward for me, or new groups of spiritual beings are presented to me, I find that things happen 2 – 3 times to get the point across and let me know that I really am not off my rocker. It will be interesting to see what comes next.

Most important of all, is that when you meet or get introduced to new energies of the light, those energies will not make you do something that is not right. They will know how to work with you in a loving way and show you what can be done. It is time for you to no longer walk in fear. If something has come into your space that is not of the light, it will cause mental anxiety, create negative chitter chatter, make you feel sick, depressed and tired and try to get you to do things that are morally wrong. You can tell this energy to leave. The following is compliments of my good friend and must be said with conviction:

"This is my body. You have no right to be here. Leave now."

Many times when the angel realm or the ancient ones are present, the feeling of love is so strong that I get tears in my eyes. The feeling is something that cannot felt unless you are open to feeling unconditional love. The love of what is, the love of God/Creator that is so strong, nothing dark can stay in its state of darkness, that dark energy is transmuted to pure love. No matter how many times I feel this love energy, that is so pure, I still cry tears of joy. We can learn to feel the essence of another's true soul. To feel another person's true soul and light is to feel pure love. This love cannot be duplicated by sexual love, partnership love. This love is unconditional with no ties to it. For years I have wondered if anyone really knows what true love is.

I feel this true love with my daughters and family. But this love can go farther, there is no judgement, no ego, only purity of God/Creator. Each and every one of us has this within. No matter what realm we come from, or physical form we inhabit. When we truly heal within, we can be pure at heart. No matter what shape or form we come in. Like the animal kingdom, even the deadliest snake can symbolize transformation, the female moose: who is extremely dangerous and protective over her young, symbolizes community and women working together. Both animals are powerful, but both have amazing energy and medicine to share, along with teaching us how to change and love all those around us.

Chapter 12

Our Thinking Patterns and What We Create....

OVER THE PREVIOUS CHAPTERS WE HAVE MENTIONED LIGHT energy and dark energy, releasing of blocks and energy imprints, and now we can really start to get into how we can create our lives for the highest good. Along with this, we need to look at our thinking patterns. What is it we can do to change things, and why do others seem to have it a lot easier?

Let's take a look at someone that we believe has it easy in life. This person seems to get whatever they want, have the home they want, the nice clothes and family. Or that person may seem to be able to get all the work they want, and no matter what they do, it always works out. Sometimes, we get jealous about these people, and envy their life style.

Let's dig a little deeper into this successful person's life. This person may have the ability to get what they want due to extremely hard work. This person may be working 50+ hours a week. This person knew what it would take to get to their goal. They did not let anything get in their way. They were the only person on their agenda, and no one else really mattered. They are determined to achieve what their heart desires or get to the places they have wanted to see. Sometimes they may even have a family and other personal responsibilities and still did really well. They believed in themselves and saw no barriers.

There can be more than what we can see from a distance. We can see their success, but do we see their health? Is it good or is it poor health? Do we see what they have missed? Do we see the time they lost with their family members? Many times there is a cost to success and it has not come as easily as we thought. Many times, people get to where they are, because they did not want to live the life they did as a child. Or were they were driven by the thought of what could happen if they became failures? Maybe they did not want to become what their parents were.

Then we look at the times when we see someone that is doing very poorly. They live in the toughest part of town. They don't have much more than what fits into their shopping cart. Too many times, we judge people and think them to be lazy and unsuccessful. Other words that I have heard over the years come to mind, but they are not nice words and only words of judgment.

Many times the outcomes of our situations are due to what our thinking patterns are. How were we raised? What was drilled into us as what was considered successful? Were we taught that we were dumb, useless, uneducated and unworthy? Do we stop ourselves because we think we are not able to achieve something? Did someone compare our success to another's?

One of the best workshops I took was "Course of Miracles". This book not only got me to see things in a different light, but it also was a huge affirmation on how my life had evolved including the personal work that I had done and work that still needed to be done. I found that I was very lucky that I had a father that did not degrade me or put me down. I realized that the lessons I learnt from my step mother were meant to be, and what I had let go of from that relationship was amazing. At the time of the workshop, I was able to see that another relationship I had with someone outside of my family was quite toxic, and I was allowing the thoughts of this person to control me energetically.

Over the last few years, I have been able to stand back and just observe and watch how people were acting in public or in family situations, watching, not saying much. If or when I did stand up and mention something when things got out of hand, my friend-ship was dropped. I was hurt at first, but later I realized that the person was still struggling with learning to be kind and gentle, and did not want to let go of what they believed as being okay and healthy patterns. Again, I will not claim to be an expert, but I lovingly let go of the friendships and connections.

We really need to look at how we view life. Are we truly happy within? Are we achieving what our hearts desire? How do we view ourselves? One of the first lessons that I learnt from the energy work, was when my friend shared "It is just a story". She did not want to hear my story that day about why I felt awful. I was hurt. But later I realized that the energy we carry with the story is what we need to let go of. If relating the story of a tragic event is causing unsettling emotions, is there something in this that we can use to learn from? Or did we use this story to become a victim? It is the same energy we carry when someone tells us we will not succeed. We have the choice to use what we hear as an advantage / dare or as a disabling label.

For example, with my step mother, I looked at the abuse as being a lesson not to harm my children. I learnt not to yell and scream or degrade my children. I also considered her own personal life, and wondered what happened when she was little. Was she physically abused? Was she verbally abused? Did she use her voice and violence to gain control of something she saw as being normal as a child or to cover her own inner pain? At an early age, I learnt to forgive her, I will never forget, but I forgave. In this way, a person can let go of unhealthy anger so not to grow into the same patterns that she showed. The odd time that I did yell at my girls, there always was an apology afterwards. I explained why I had yelled and that I did not like doing it.

With this, we can let go of what has happened to us during our life time and use the information as a learning tool, and a way to grow even more so. I was able to raise my daughters with love and compassion, and like my dad, still be there for them, no matter what. On those days when I wondered if I was a good mom, the thoughts brought awareness that I truly cared and did not want to fall into something that I was shown as a child.

Another example is when I was living in a town house in the city, a single parent of 2 children. When they were quite young, during the evening I finished off my grade 12 by completing 2 courses to get the credits I needed, in order to go to college. I was determined to provide a better life for my children and get a job that utilized my brain and analytical side. It took a lot of self-counseling and back patting to get the 2 years of Business Administration done at SAIT in Calgary. I was the oldest student at the age of 27, but I was very determined to go far with this. I complete the 2 years and obtained the courses that I needed for accounting. This determination built my self-worth and it also inspired friends that were around me. This education was something that I wanted to do, and to this day, do not regret.

When I got married the second time, I was the office manager and book-keeper for my husband's business for over 7 years. I succeeded at pretty much anything I tried and got past any childhood trauma.

Even though, there were times over the 2 years when people tried to discourage me, such as college instructors, my ex-partner, and other family members, I kept on going. I achieved my goal. The first year at SAIT was tough, but after I had got past the first hurdles, it got easier, and I did really well. There was an instructor that was very demeaning towards females, and I made sure I passed his class, barely. In the next math class with a different instructor, I got an A in the math. I used the first instructor's unkind words as a personal dare. This is what I see as being part of our thinking patterns, seeing past what we are told, and going beyond any boundary that may pop up, and not letting others put you down.

After finishing college, I started to work as a bookkeeper in Calgary. Part of me was very lonely, being a single parent, I was a wee bit depressed, yet I was still determined. I remember looking out the window, washing dishes and visualizing being in a house that was mine, with a partner and lots of gardens to play in. I held onto that vision. I held this dream in my heart. Most of the activities I did with my girls were outside: playing in the parks, going for walks, camping, doing crafts and enjoying life. We made the best of what we had. We laughed, loved, hugged and supported each other.

About 5 years later, we lived in a house in Cochrane with a huge yard, and I was remarried. I created many new gardens, and the town became home to my girls, even though they were a bit annoyed that they had to leave their school buddies behind. That vision is what I held onto. That thought of achieving what my heart really loved to do, earning a good living and being outside and working in the gardens in my free time.

Even though I had the odd sad thought, I remembered that I needed to create better thinking patterns for myself; I needed to go beyond what others tried to deter me from. When you take the time to stop the old, unhealthy thoughts from controlling you, you can live a very healthy life. Good health is a state of wealth in itself.

I was introduced to a family that grew up on very little. The mother was a drinker, who was never at home, and the children raised themselves. They did have a lot of help from other family members. They were taught that good things were only for the rich and that they did not deserve or could have what others had. That this state of low esteem was normal and that they could not do anything about it. One of the children met someone that showed this person how far she could go, if she worked for it and learnt to believe that she was much better than what she had been taught. Today, that lady owns a house, has a family of her own, and is very proud of where she has gotten. Someone believed in her. Someone knew how to push this person a bit farther and encourage her. This lady's sibling is still struggling.

When we believe that we cannot have something, or that we will always be stuck, or that we are not capable of doing something, the energy we create will be that. We really do start to live that life. A person is able to overcome that obstacle when they are ready or have had enough. But this takes a lot of determination. Many times we can do this on our own, but sometimes we will seek outside help. If we don't make those changes, then our life will continue that way. When I am looking for changes in my life, I always ask for my highest good.

Our highest good or soul can lead us down pathways that we may never have seen, as our vision may have been clouded by doubt or low self-worth. Even if we get a glimpse of something, that glimpse is a sign of what we can do. Our highest good or soul knows what our gifts are and what we are truly capable of. When we get an idea and get a truth shiver, or divine intervention, where we start to cry happy tears, this is an indication of what is possible. Sometimes we don't quite see the whole picture, as we need to start at the beginning and enjoy the journey and learning. This is what I did with the holistic healing.

We need to learn how to love ourselves for who we are and love ourselves so that we do not bring disharmony into our homes and lives. This love can help to dissolve any worries that we hold onto. This love helps us to enjoy life to its fullest. This love will not harm others around us and will not create chaos and hardship. When we see or observe others and see the disharmony, we can show compassion, but we will not be pulled into what is going on. Love overcomes disharmony.

Disharmony is created by unhealthy thinking patterns. We also need to learn that we do not need to get pulled into someone else's drama and stories. Disharmony is what creates judgment, criticalness of ourselves and others. It also leads to unfair observations, such as thinking that the wealthy person has it better or that the poor person is lazy. We all have our own journey. Maybe the financially wealthy person, is unhealthy and sad, or maybe they truly are happy, as they overcame the obstacles of unhealthy thinking and life as a child. Maybe the poor person is truly happy within, with very few responsibilities, able to travel at a whim, and comfortable in their surroundings. Or maybe that poor person is poor because of physical and mental abuse as a child. Maybe they were severely injured and did not get the support they needed to heal on all levels.

There have been many times when I have felt that others were intimidated by me. They will act like I lack intelligence and will tell me how things should be done. They take on a sense of superiority and find a way to let me go, whether it is a job or a friendship. They see something in me that I don't pay attention to. Many times after leaving a job I get feedback from the other employees and they know about how unfair the layoff was, as my work exceeded what was expected and I outshone the supervisor and I was honest. These were times when I needed encouragement, not to be let down. This has happened with many friends and clients. They hold themselves back due to the stories they were told by others who did not want them to shine and be successful.

As this chapter was unfolding, I saw where it was to lead to. We need to sit back when we hear someone putting us down. We need to look at where that person has been and what they have done to bring changes to their lives, before we take to heart what they are saying. Many times when people lash out at others, it is a reflection of their own lives. If someone tells you to cut your hair, or stop drawing, or that you cannot sing, what are they really saying? Did someone else tell them that they could not do these things? A friend would encourage you to draw, even if they believe they are better, or if they are scared you are a better artist than they are.

When we step away from expectations that we believe are placed on us, we can do amazing things with our lives.

At this time in my life others may believe that I don't do real work with real responsibilities, as I don't work full time in an 8 – 5 job. I have a home, I am able to get out for a lot of walks during my work day and my days off can be in the middle of the week. I don't wear designer clothes, I live a simple life and I get to teach weird things like crystal healing, Reiki and reflexology. I am very rich within. My health is amazing, considering I was in a head-on collision 2 months ago on the highway. The work and crafts I do for a living has my heart singing. I love life, I work honestly, I am humble, I love talking to the birds and squirrels and I am there for others when they need help. I laugh, play, sing, dance and love life.

This has all come into play as I have learnt how to look after myself and the space that I live in. I have learned how to censor my thinking, to meditate, to let go and protect my well-being. Next, we will go into how we can set boundaries and protect ourselves so that we all can live life in abundance on all levels.

When we let go of what others try to lead us into believing, we can create a healthier life. We just need to remember not to hold onto the energy of someone else's harmful words and beliefs. We need to remember that someone else's reality may not be the same as our own. We also need to remember not to impose our beliefs on others. We can gently share a little bit of what we are interested in. Be kind and gentle in our words, thoughts and be in the heart centre.

Chapter 13

Protecting Our Space

A LOT OF THE TRAINING OVER THE YEARS INVOLVED LEARNING how to provide protection for our bodies: physically, mentally, emotionally and spiritually. I found that many students went to other workshops and did not learn how to cut cords, or how to recognize when something around them was being afflicted by their own anger or someone else's anger. They were surprised what they ended up learning, as I was sharing what needed to be learnt by each group. Each group brought something different to the table.

When we pay attention to what is happening to our bodies, or space at home and work, we can create a healthier sense of well-being without having to try to change others. We just need to focus on what we are willing to accept around us. If our bodies or our space feel heavy, or we are hurting, what is it that we need to change? What is it that we need to let go of or say no to.

Feeling and listening are the greatest tools that we have to rec-ognize if something is not right. This is using our intuition. There have been many times that things were drawn to my attention that I should have listened to, and the result sure became a huge lesson.

Sometimes, even though we may have cut a cord or distanced ourselves from someone, they may still try to energetically harm us. This is what I call a psychic attack. When someone sends unhealthy energy into your space because they are uncomfort-able with you or blaming you for something that happened that was their own doing, you become their scapegoat. Sometimes we don't realize that this has happened till years later. Something can happen in a previous life, where something was thrown at us, or done to us (no matter how we received the energy). If we were not able to heal this situation, we could carry this with us. The lives following will experience setbacks or beliefs about why we become sick or have not succeeded at what we pursue as a living. When we become more sensitive to our bodies, we can pick up things a lot faster and recognize what is truly going on.

First, we will look at some of the things that can occur in our space and the ways it can affect our health on all levels. A lot of this is going on, whether we like it or not. For many years, I tried to hide from the fact that people can actually do these things or that these things are carried from lifetime to lifetime.

Anger darts

Anger Darts are created by someone throwing anger towards you, and it does not matter how the anger was triggered. It could be from something you did, or someone that someone thought you did. These anger darts feel like energetic darts hitting you all over the back or at a particular part of the body that it they were sent to. We need to be very careful how we project images, thoughts or feelings. It is wrong to throw any sort of anger at anyone or anything. We can hold onto this anger that was thrown at us from years ago or from past lives.

I have felt this happen. I had someone throw anger darts at me just over a year ago in the early spring of 2014. First lesson was to experience this and be aware of it. For about 2 years, I had been observing a previous friend talk about anger spears, throwing energy and hissing at people. I found these actions quite disturbing and a few times stopped this person from doing this to other people.

Right before the anger darts were thrown, I was hoping for the best for a person that I had just seen on a walk with my granddaughter, and I sent best wishes to another person at the same time. I knew within that both were going through something that was not easy and asked that they be helped out for their highest good. After I had passed this person and was about a block away, I felt a whole bunch of energetic darts hit my back. It did not really hurt, but right away I knew what happened. I wondered what was going on, and why, and I wondered where they came from. I had a strong feeling that this was connected to the person that I was sharing good wishes for. I tried to send these darts back with love and compassion. With this I learnt that I needed to bring in the white healing energies to dissolve the effect of the anger darts, nothing more.

When confronting this person later on, she pretended to not know what happened. I just asked why she did not call me for help instead of doing what she did. She denied it, and said she felt so much anger from me when we had seen each other at a coffee shop about 2 months previous to the attack. What she felt was all of the anger that was brought to me from other people that had encounters with her. I never said anything bad about her, and only let these friends share what they felt in a safe space. When we saw each other at the coffee shop, it triggered the memory of what others had said. That is the anger that she felt, and maybe a bit of mine, wondering how she could make others so mad. I did rudely scold her after the accident, and I shared that she should have called me and talked to me instead of throwing anger darts. I asked why she did not stop to help me out and her reply was if she had, I would have thought it was her that did this. I giggled to myself, as I knew she was lying to me. In order to protect myself better, I was to recognize that if something like this happened again, I could just bring in Gods healing light to dissolve the energy of the impact, ask for forgiveness and healing for both myself and the other person, nothing more. I realized that this could happen again, but now I knew how to react in a better way and protect my body from absorbing the negativity. I also realized that I should not have allowed all that anger from my friends be shown to this person. Or maybe this was meant to happen so that we both learnt what happens when we project our feelings that strongly.

Recommended Solutions:

1. Bring in the white light to help heal the energy that was created from the anger darts.

2. Ask for forgiveness for both yourself and the other person, regardless of the role you played in a situation. Sometimes we are just the scape goat for someone's anger of not achieving what they want.

Sometimes we are receiving back what we put out.

3. Learn how to communicate and share when you are getting unhappy feedback or reports.

4. Perform a good smudging when you get home or ask for blessings and healing for both parties.

Resentment or anger swords

Resentment or anger swords are created by someone that wants to stop you in your tracks. They may resent what they think you have or have accomplished, and they don't want you to go any farther. This person might not have the same beliefs or they might want you to fall back so that they can be the first in line for a promotion, or be the recipient of a better life. Or they may even be mad because you finally stood up to them. This energy does feel like a sword in the back. I have seen this energetically on many clients, especially in healers from past lives.

Sometimes these swords were even from past partners in those lives or others from battle. The swords could have been either energy swords or real swords and the imprints of this action stayed along the soul line throughout the past lives and present life.

I had a clearing done for me about 3 years ago, and someone had sent an anger sword when I was in my mid-twenties. I was not sure what this really felt like (other than what I saw with clients) until a few months ago. I had started my walk on a nice day, all alone, and by the time I was half way back home, I felt a discomfort in my right shoulder blade. This felt like a sword, similar to what I have seen in clients from past life experiences. It felt like a pain in the back, along the shoulder blade. It did not feel like sore muscles but more like an unwanted discomfort, a sharp pain. With the clients, most of the swords were from anger swords that were caused by actual swords that caused a death. When I felt this sword in my back, I asked where it came from. Right away I was shown a vision of a friend that I just let go of. Over the 2–3 year friendship, I found that I needed a lot of patience and compassion. This is an awesome person that I got to enjoy many good adventures with but the friendship ended due to standing up for myself and saying no. It was another lesson, but one from which I knew I could shift really quickly. I was able to energetically draw out the sword and put a protective dome around me.

Recommended Solutions:

1. Infuse them with healing light, and then gently extract the sword. I always ask Archangel Michael to bag the energy sword and escort it out.

2. Learn how to close doors and cut cords when a friendship has ended. Again we ask for Archangel Michael's assistance to do the cord cutting and Archangel Raphael to assist in sealing the area of the cord for both parties.

3. Ask for healing for both parties and keep that door closed until the other person is ready to fully accept responsibility for their actions.

Contracts/Curses

Contracts are another way of putting up barriers for someone or our self from previous lives or present life, with or without our consent. I truly don't believe that all contracts are made for the highest good of a soul. These contracts can inhibit a person from living their next life to the fullest. The contract can also cause a lot of resentment and hardship in the next life. Curses can have the same effect. Curses can inhibit a person and create sickness, financial loss, family disruptions and more.

A contract that came to mind affected a close friend that had, in a previous life, gone through a lot of discomfort while being raised. The mother of this person did not protect the child and the child swore not to have children in her next life. She placed a contract on herself, not realizing the impact that it would carry forward.

There are contracts that are unknowingly placed on our lives by other beings so that we come back in our next life and submit to extreme fighting, forced labour and slavery. These contracts are unethical and can be removed. These contracts only serve those that placed them. The person that is contracted goes through a really tough and restricted life. Their soul is not able to achieve what it desires or is capable of.

Last week, I was presented with a person that believed something had been energetically following him for several years. While working on him, I mentioned something about black magic, as I had really not seen much of this stuff and was very leery of asking. He replied that he lived in an area where there was a lot of black and white magic. Curses were being placed by the black magic, and then a white magic healer would have to remove the curse. If you were unaware of the curse, it could take several years for it to register. With this person, the curse was energetically connected to his lower back.

Recommended Solutions:

1. With contracts and curses I found that you need to sternly void them and state that fact that they are non renewable.

2. While doing this we can send unconditional love in the direction of the source from which the energy came from. I would also do a cord cutting for this other person, whether you know them or not.

Implants

Alien implants are physical or energetic objects placed in someone's body after they have been abducted by an alien. This can even happen in a dream state to warn someone that someone else may be trying to control their life. The purpose of these implants range from tracking a person to mind control. This is something that conspiracy theorists claim has been happening for years. During the clearing done for me, 3 years ago, the healer removed an implant that was placed in my third eye chakra. This inhibited me from fully opening to the other realms and insights. It also created a criticism that affected the way I saw things.

Recommended Solutions:

1. Seek a healer to help you remove the implant, the same as you would for contracts and curses.

2. Be careful of what you want to happen in your next life. I always ask for my highest good, no matter what that looks like. We cannot control someone else's life.

Entities, parasites, argons

Entities are usually hanging around the lower leg area and can be picked up anywhere. They are recognized by a sick feeling one you get when being around a higher energy such as crystals. These entities can be created by heavy thinking, excessive use of drugs and alcohol.

Parasites usually attach to the back or arm area, and attach with a hook-like connection. I have heard of a 2 prong hook parasite and of one that attaches with just one hook. Parasites are harder to disconnect and can cause a lot of anger in the person, depression and a feeling of being really tired. The parasite absorbs all the good energy from a person and can leave them feeling out of sorts. One friend noticed the one attached to her within the week, and it had left 2 marks on her back from the hooks. The marks did go away a few days after the Reiki session. These can be picked up just about anywhere, but more so with old artifacts or practices of unhealthy lifestyles. The second friend had one tag along with her for several years till another healer saw it tagging along behind her.

Argons are usually attached to the back of their host. The argons love to suck in negative energy and thrive on it. They get bigger as they suck up the heavy energy around them. An argon can interfere with a person's intuition and energy. They can also create a very sore back for the host. I had a student come in for a Reiki class with one attached to him. At first, I thought that he just had a sore back. One of the other students observed this fellow's shirt moving back and forth when he was doing Reiki on another student. Later in the afternoon, while I watched the students I saw the same thing. There was no way that his shirt could move in and out like that. At first, being a bit nervous, I asked the energy to leave. It was like he had a monkey on his back. Within a few minutes, I had to bring in the pure healing energy and dissolve the argon till Archangel Michael could escort it out safely. After this, the students back did not hurt and his intuition accelerated. I kept the fellows after the class to do a full clearing for both of them.

Recommended solutions:

1. Don't try to pull one off, it could hurt the host and will try to hold on even tighter. Entities, parasites and argons need to be infused with pure healing light and love to enable them to let go.

2. Ensure the entity, parasite or argon is safely escorted out, and then you must do healing work for the imprint that may have been left behind from the heavy energy being.

3. Pay attention to where you go. If you find that your energy has greatly shifted, and you are not your normal, happy self, do a really good smudging with sage and work with crystals like selenite, kyanite and tourmaline. If your work is required in areas that are similar to bars and pubs, keep one or more of these crystals on you while you are working for better protection. I have even done this for going to drum circles and health expos.

Lost or Unhappy Spirits

Lost spirits don't always attach because of what energy state you are in. They may do one of 2 things; attach to you because they know you will take them out of the surroundings that they have been stuck in or they will invite themselves into your space. Lost spirits are spirits from people that did not cross over to the other side, as they thought God would not accept them. They will befriend the vulnerable, who are open to the spirit world and are lonely or unhappy with their lives. The lost spirit has made unhealthy choices in its life times and caused unnecessary chaos that was damaging for those around them. As the spirit goes from life to life, it gets darker due to thinking that it cannot change what they have done. This is the unhealthy ego state of the spirit and it has a hard time going back to being a beautiful loving soul. The energy from the lost spirit can make one feel depressed, sick to the stomach and unsure with your life. When I have worked on someone with a very lost spirit attached, I can feel the fear, and I feel like I want to throw up.

An unhappy spirit is one that has been stuck to the earth plane due to the way the spirit/soul was raised. Again, like earlier in the book, I mentioned how people have been taught that they will not go to heaven if they had sex without being married, or did other so-called unhealthy things that were deemed bad due to strict belief systems. When these people pass away their spirits may stay along the road side, in their homes or in the area of death. Sometimes, spirits will linger behind because a family member will not let them go. If the family member is still alive, the spirit will show up with them. Or we may find them in a home that someone moved in. At first when a family moves in, the spirit is okay, but over time the spirit gets agitated and starts acting out. It is unhappy because it can no longer laugh, play, make love, be heard or eat like a human. This unhappy spirit can cause depression, an uneasy feeling when entering a certain room, or it may even start breaking things in the home.

Recommended Solutions:

1. With both the lost spirit and unhappy spirit, one must be strong and fully in the heart centre. One must remember that pure love is stronger than any heavier energy and the God / Creator will be with us as they help the spirits to shift their frequency.

2. Once the spirit has shifted in energy I ask Archangel Michael and his team to assist with the cord cutting and to safely escort them out for further processing.

3. We do further energy work to help dissolve and heal any imprint from the spirit that may have been left behind.

Demon energy

Demon energy is strong, and it can cause chaos and not allow you to make changes in your life. It hinders healthier thoughts and stops you from living life to the fullest. When there is a demon energy residing within someone, you can see a flicker of the red eyes. I first saw this energy or the red eyes, in a picture that a gal sent to me of her friend. We knew right away what it was. There was the demon dog that had come into my home with the renter a year ago (a few months after I saw the picture). I saw the outline of the dog on my stairs, and what really stood out were the red eyes. The demon dog was created by the excessive use of drugs and alcohol. People do not realize that whether they are or not, open to the spirit realm, when they engage in over use of cannabis, heroin, cocaine, the darker energies will come into their space. This energy can cause fear and lack of judgement even when the person is not indulging. With this demon energy, there is no compassion for others: there is no self-worth, it is like being dead with no healthy spirit left at all.

This energy can also be brought in by practicing what one calls the dark arts. To create potions or spells for one's personal gain or for another's gain at the cost of someone else's highest good. When we try to obtain something or control something at the cost of someone else's life and wellbeing we create a disharmony and unease that is against another's best interest. All love is gone, the light has gone out.

Recommended Solutions:

1. Avoid going into fear mode. This energy is a bit harder to work with for the beginner, fear will enhance or strengthen the demon energy. We need to go fully into the heart centre and work with Gods pure love and light. We need to know that this love and light is extremely strong and will make the changes required. When this is being done, you must be of clear energy, in the state of full love and very strong, knowing and letting the energy know that its time is done.

2. Ask Archangel Michael to assist and help escort the energy safely out. I am not sure if the energy goes to purgatory (a for ever jail like state) or for further processing to assist the energy to make changes for a healthier state of well-being.

3. Smudge the person or area fully smudged afterwards with white sage (the thick buffalo sage is a lot stronger than wild sage) and the vibration of the person or area needs to be brought up with the white light to create less chance of this happening again.

Caution: You need to be careful when working with the dark energies such as the demon and greys, as this is not a game. You will need to ask for help from the angel realm and ancient ones and work together as a team.

Greys

Greys appear to be an automated, thoughtless, senseless, controlling being with absolutely no love or compassion. I am not sure of how they originated and don't know if they can energetically change. The greys appear cloaked. I could not see a face, only a shape like a human with a dark grey cloak. With one person, I felt an electrical charge come from them, when I attempted to show the friend a new technique I had learnt. This person did not know that the grey was residing in their space. But what the person realized later, was that the greys create a heavy negative chitter chatter in the mind. This can be the same for dark spirits and demon energies. They try to interfere with our thinking process and don't like the positive thinking of love and light. Greys are very controlling and want to dominate your space and life just like the dark spirits. But the difference is a dark spirit can change back to love and light, and I don't think the greys can do this, but I could be wrong on this one.

Recommended Solutions:

1. Avoid going into fear mode. Again, this energy is a bit harder to work with for the beginner, fear can enhance or strengthen the grey energy. You need to go fully into the heart centre and work with Gods pure love and light. You need to be very persistent and demand that the grey exit the body of the human.

2. Ask Archangel Michael and his team to assist and help escort the energy safely out. The greys are sent to a place of no return. The greys serve no purpose to those in either the light or dark and they do what they want for their own selfish needs.

3. Smudge the person or area fully afterwards with white sage (the thick buffalo sage is a lot stronger than wild sage) and the vibration of the person or area needs to be brought up with the

white light to create less chance of this happening again. I would fully suggest a full light body integration for the person.

Caution: You need to be careful when working with the greys and dark energies, this is not a game. You need to ask for help from the angel realm and ancient ones and work together as a team. When these energies are not properly worked with they will return and cause chaos somewhere else. That is not want you want. You want a loving place to live in.

Cord cutting

This is a method to help release you from people and places that could be inhibiting you from going forward. You can do cord cutting from unhealthy relationships whether they are with family, friends or past friends and partners. Cord cutting is also useful if you are trying to sell a house, or keep getting pulled back to something that is unhealthy or no longer required in your life. This is very important for all of us, and a must for those who work in the health services field: doctors, nurses, holistic practitioners and counsellors.

Partnerships

When you connect as a partner, you in a sense can become one. This is good during intimate times, but it is not healthy if on a daily basis. When a couple becomes so attached to each other, the relationship becomes unhealthy and each one relies too much on the other. When one person is dominating the relationship, the other person is not given any room to grow. Many times there is restrictive upbringing and ideals or domestic abuse involved in this. In each relationship, you should be able to fully pursue your own dreams while still being able to enjoy the presence of a partner.

1. It is okay to energetically connect, but if one partner is the domineering partner, you need to cut the cord whether you are living with the partner or living apart from each other. The more

you practice this, the stronger you get till you can figure out if the relationship is worth pursuing.

2. If there is domestic abuse, it is time to consider outside help. I have also seen it where one would say they are being abused, but are the abuser themselves. Sometimes this can be a mirror of our own actions. If you are being abused, please seek outside support.

3. When you do chord cutting from a partner you truly love, you can start to find your own interests and talents beyond what your partner is doing. Many times, partners can lead healthy and productive lives working together, but each needs their own responsibilities and time.

Parent and young adult

When a parent holds onto a child too tightly, especially after they have reached the age of 18, the parent's tight hold can hinder the child from growing and being successful. Only a very strong willed child would be able to succeed. When our children reach the age of 18 and are done school, our job is over. It is up to the child to grow, to learn and to explore beyond the reach of the parent. We can offer encouragement when needed, and pray for the best for them, no matter what the outcome looks like. Maybe it is the path of the child to have a hard adult life, maybe it is the path for them to succeed at something we may never have considered. This is their journey. This is where cord cutting can be helpful for both parent and young adult. If we worry too much and don't let go, the young adult can get sick too.

Recommended Solutions:

1. Let the young adult pursue the path of their dreams.

2. Do not encourage the young adult to be unproductive, and not work for a living. We all need to contribute one way or another.

3. The young adult must take responsibility for their actions, not you.

Friends and family

Friends and family are a big part of our lives and upbringing. We can have some very wonderful people around us as we grow up. Yet as we get older, some of the friendships diminish, or we see less of our relatives. People can come and go. Some friendships last a really long time, and some are short. Each person has their own journey and many times their own interests. This can happen with our own children, sisters and brothers, cousins and close friends.

There is a lot of disharmony in families due to religious beliefs, personal upbringing or strict control and manipulation. We need to honor each person for their own journey and what they are doing. But we also need to let go of those who do not support our interests. If we are living a healthy and vibrant life, no excessive alcohol or drugs, eating well, and good state of emotional well-being, we deserve to have the space to do it in. If someone is not supporting this, then the relationship will either fade away or it will require cord cutting.

Recommended Solutions:

1. Many times we need to let go of family or friends that will not support us or try to dominate the friendship. Friendships should be based on shared interests, not control. The same applies to family.

2. We need to listen to each other and not try to make someone else believe what we do.

Work environments

When we go home at night from work we need to detach from that space and those involved. This also applies to doctors, nurses, holistic practitioners and counsellors. Our bodies need rest, and proper nourishment to be able to function on a healthy level. If we bring this home with us, we will still be tired the next day. With those in the health services, we need to detach from the outcome of whatever service we provided that day. When we work from the heart, and have done our best, it is up to the recipient to take this forward for themselves. We cannot stay attached to our clients, and those that we encountered during the day.

Recommended Solutions:

1. Over the years, as I learnt to let go of what goes on in other's lives, my own life become more peaceful and healthier. I had less worry, fewer sick stomachs, and fewer headaches. I leave work there.

2. When you walk out the door of work, try cord cutting or closing an internal door, this will be explained below.

Property

I have done clearings and cord cutting for properties, as the new owners were not able to go ahead with renovations. People can create energetic attachments to property they lived on, and didn't want to let go of. An acreage I worked with had a previous renter's attachment that felt like strong anger. When we first drove up to the property, it felt like the cattle there were really mad and not happy with their home. I thought it weird at first, but when we left, my friend noticed a huge change in the energy of the cattle. When we are getting ready to move, whether we like it or not, we need to let go of what was so that we can start a new life somewhere else. We need to cut the cord with the property, for ourselves and all our family members and relations that may have an interest in the property.

Recommended Solutions:

1. Do the cord cutting when you know you need to leave a place.

2. Do the cord cutting for all the family.

3. Bless the property and land for the new residents.

Cord cutting methods:

1. I still will ask Archangel Michael to help assist with cord cutting when I know there is a deeper connection that I am not aware of. I will ask for Archangel Raphael to assist with sealing in the area of the cords. I ask this to be done for both me and the other person or property.

2. With the Reiki training, I learnt about using the Raku Symbol for cord cutting. I will use this symbol and intention of the action after each phone call, after each client and with family members.

3. Closing doors is like a cord cutting. I have learnt to use the door for relationships, both friends and family. There is a time when we again need to protect our space. Sometimes this action feels stronger when I do not want to reconnect on any level with the other person until I have seen a huge shift. I visualize a door being closed and locked, with the other person on the other side of the door. Within minutes, I can feel that closure.

Other ways of protecting our space and home

Learning to protect my space was something that needed to be learned over the years and after finding several ways of looking after my space or the space that I am about to enter, my well-being has greatly improved. I am an early indigo that has had many of the experiences that the indigo and crystal children are having now. Some experiences were fun learning about and had me giggling, and some of them were downright scary. What we will do is look at all the situations that come to mind. Please remember that what works with the kids also works with the adults.

Our home

As was mentioned earlier in the book, our home needs to have clear and happy energy for the family unit to do well. Some members are really sensitive, and others could not care less. So we are working for the one whose physical, mental, emotional and spiritual well-being is assaulted by chaos and unwanted visitors. When someone comes into my home and is not vibrating in the heart centre along with having ill health or depression, the sage will come out right after they leave. If we don't do this, the energy will linger and affect those that are still in the house. Just now, several memories came to mind where I unknowingly allowed something to linger or happen, and others around me were greatly affected. I would not be surprised if they walked away with stories. The last time that I can remember this happening was over 14 years ago.

Several years ago, someone dropped by for a visit. After they had left and I went down stairs, the welcome sign that was on the wall by the front door fell to the ground and broke. I believe that this person was heartbroken, as she did not receive the welcome that she had expected. I started to do energy work on the main floor to dispel the sadness and disappointment. Today, we are really good friends again.

Someone came to do some plumbing in the house, and this person was angry and frustrated. It felt horrid, I took the granddaughter for a walk, and about a block away, I realized the difference in the energy from the house to being outside. This started my journey of finding ways to keep spaces in better harmony.

Recommended Solutions:

1. Smudging with sage: For a fresh start, whether you are moving into a home, or living in a house that was newly built, the home needs to be thoroughly smudged with sage and blessed with sweet-grass or lavender. One starts this by smudging clockwise from the basement to the top flooring. (You need to be fully present in the heart center, bringing in Archangel Michael for help.)

First go around with sage, then for the second round with the sweet-grass and lavender. If you are still having a hard time, and the energy is not shifting, it is suggested to call in someone that has had experience with this and knows how to release and heal any of the imprints of emotions and events that have left a heavy feeling. An expert can also assist with safely escorting out any lingering spirits. This is something that takes practice, and I know within that everyone can learn to do this. The secret is not to be in fear, and yet not be cocky.

2. Working with crystals: We can use crystals for several things including setting grids around the property, the house, or even individual rooms. When we set grids, it is for the highest good of the home and for protection and good health.

Property: I have walked clockwise around my property and sprinkled selenite shards and pieces to protect the land. Or you can walk clockwise and set a protective crystal in each corner of the property.

House: with the house, you can again go clockwise and place a protective crystal in each corner of the home. One can even use a wand to energetically draw a protective wall from crystal to crystal till each wall is done. North, east, south, west and then back to the north.

Rooms: Each room can be done with crystals that the individual needs for their well-being at that time. Amethyst would be perfect for each room, as it heals on all levels. Or you may need more rose quartz for the heart, or tourmaline for those who have bad dreams. Again, place a crystal in each corner or under the bed of the person residing in that room.

3. Working with oils and herbs: You can use essential oils in your home, such as lavender or sage and there are many more that provide assistance during colds, flu or depression. Some of the oils can be used to bring up the vibration of your home.

4. Working with energy and angels: When my home feels not right and no matter what I have tried, I ask for assistance from the angels, fairies, and those of the light, and go into Reiki mode to bring in positive energy to help with the shifting.

Personal space

Our personal space can be wherever we are at the time, or in our home. Each individual has their own stuff going on. It is an honour to see someone that is fully care free and has no worries. It appears as if they are walking in heaven at all times while still in a human body. This is a motto that I share on my website and in daily life, "bringing heaven to earth." When we are able to achieve this, life can be enjoyed to the fullest. We can enjoy going to school as a kid or adult. We can travel safely (physically and emotionally), and we can reside in a comfortable space at home and fully relax.

Over the last couple of years, I have had several mothers come over with their sons. The boys were from between the ages of 8 to 10. They too, like females, go through a growing spree and hormonal change of some sort. They become more sensitive, and the psychic abilities starting to blossom. But when the mother and child don't know what is happening, the child gets sick, and does not want to go to school, does not want to go to bed at night as they are scared or nervous. This also applies to young girls going into puberty. Both girls and boys are becoming quite empathic and others may think of them as just being crazy and want them to go through testing, counselling, and more. This also applies to adults. When we, the empaths can learn how to protect ourselves, we can have more fun without being on guard at all times.

Recommend Suggestions: For adults and children

1. Smudging with sage: We cannot smudge in the schools and parks, but a good clearing with sage in the home can help. If you come home and are really shaken from an event (I will wake up the next day with a hang-over feeling, and I don't drink), you can smudge your body from top to bottom. I use a feather to bring the smoke closer to the person. Or I will use the sage smudge in my bedroom, going around the room with it and over my body after a bad dream if I feel really shaken by the dream.

2. Working with crystals: Crystals can be used for so many things. The kids and even I at age 55, can wear a piece of kyanite, or have the kyanite in our pockets, purses, backpacks. I have suggested this to many mothers, and they came back with wonderful feedback on the positive results. I now have a piece of selenite in a small bag in my pillow case at night. The bad dreams are lessening, and I am sleeping a lot better. As an empath, we can pick up on each other's bad dreams and energies at night too. The selenite may be too strong for some of the kids. We can also

teach the kids to do happy grids in their bedrooms. With one fellow, after doing some energy work on him and sharing a bit on doing grids, his whole well-being shifted over the weekend and within 2 days this fellow went from being scared to being very proud and vibrant. He also learnt to protect his space with the crystals. I make sure the kyanite and tourmaline are on me when I am in big crowds and busy buildings.

3. Working with oils and herbs: There are several essential oils that can be used on a daily basis. There are oils to help you sleep, to focus, or for more self-confidence. Lavender helps me to sleep when the global energy is strong and unwell. Rescue remedy is a herbal tincture that helps me transition from one place to another. There are oils that can help both kids and adults focus better, so that they are not distracted by other energies around them. This can be really helpful for those attending school and college.

4. Working with energy and angels: We can use energy such as Reiki energy to help us when we pick up on other people's emotions or physical discomforts. (Eg: Once while traveling into the city with a friend, when we came to a certain district, I started to feel really sick, like I wanted to throw up and my bowels were being affected too. Right away I went into Reiki mode. Within about 10 minutes I felt a lot better and was able to enjoy the rest of my day.) I also ask the angels to travel or be with me when I am nervous about going somewhere. Or I ask them to be with my children and grandchildren.

All of the above advice for the personal space, can be applied no matter where we go, except the use of the burning sage. You could wear a sage essential oil or do energy work for the area that you intend to be in.

Chapter 14

Conclusion to Changing and Healing Our Lives, Spirit and Soul

IT IS FITTING THAT WE STOP AT CHAPTER 14. 1+4=5. NUMERICALLY the number 5 means to transform, to change, alchemy. Something in your life is to change for the better. My house address for over 20 years was 221 = 5. Years in this home brought many changes and learning, not only for myself and my family, but also for clients and students of the workshops that were taught here.

This book is not meant to scare anyone, but to bring awareness to what is really going on in the world around us. All things on this planet have an energetic vibration to them, humans, animals, soil, houses, furniture, mountains, lakes and rivers, the air we breathe in, and the roads and land we travel on. I am hoping this information will help you on your journey. You are not alone.

We all are connected energetically and can receive some amazing and life-changing messages. Our bodies, our minds, those around us whether alive, in human form, in animal form or in the spirit realm are all able to heal, physically, mentally, emotionally and spiritually. We can heal our past lives and our present life.

I truly believe that we can heal our bodies to the point where we can lead healthy and vibrant lives. Yes, you may have to take the odd medication, say, for diabetes, or vitamins and minerals to keep your chemical state in balance. Or maybe you are taking a medication to help out with the heart. There are some really good medications that have been created by the pharmaceuticals. But there are many medications that can cause a lot of harm when not used properly or tested properly. I truly believe that our real medicine is in the food we eat that is created on this planet. We all can learn how to use Divine Life Energy to release and heal the blocks that we hold on to.

I am really hoping that this book will help with those that have not quite believed what they were taught. I pray that those that were told that they were crazy or are really sensitive because of what they hear or feel will read this too. We are not crazy. We just need to learn to slow down the information that we are receiving internally and externally along with learning how to filter some of it. We all have amazing abilities that have been dismissed or numbed by drugs.

It is up to you to find ways that work for you. What has been suggested in this book is not the law but rather suggestions for what has worked for me and others around me. I needed to try different things till I felt comfortable with what was working. Be kind and gentle with yourself and know with time and practice all will fall into place till you are able to create that comfortable life that you truly deserve.

I keep at the back of my mind that, even though I see really weird stuff and hear weird things, the work that I am meant to do is being brought to me in a different way. I don't have to fill out a resume I just listen to God and the beings of the light to bring forth love and light onto this beautiful planet called Mother Earth. We can be the healers for Mother Earth and her inhabitants along with helping with healing the spirit realm. I am also very grateful for all the sisters and brothers that join me on this journey.

Please remember that if you do receive too much information, or hear too many voices, or get negative chitter, ask to have all of this toned down for you. When I started practicing more with the psychic work, I asked to only be shown what I needed to see or hear. I did not want to hear other peoples' thoughts all the time. I did not want to be probing into other peoples' minds, and I did not want to see things that were irrelevant to another person's healing or life. What I am shown is for the highest good.

I am going to leave you with some questions and things to ponder on. Hopefully most of your questions have been answered for you. We all just need to listen. We all can be really healthy on all levels.

What is it that you are willing to do to get to your goals?

Is your body getting sore? What is it telling you?

What message do you keep getting, over and over on something that you could do and don't think you are capable of doing?

How many voices do you keep hearing within? Are the voices nice? Are the voices mean and nasty? Have you set boundaries?

Are you following your dreams? Are you allowing the dreams to go beyond your expectations?

Are you keeping your space safer and living with a positive state of mind?

**You are a beautiful amazing soul that just
needed to be recognized by you!**

Sending lots of love, light and blessings for all of your journeys.

PS:

On a 7 day I did my 1st written channelling.

On a 7 day I sent payment to get my book printed.

**Chapter 7 was about the truth about spirits
and why I was writing the book.**

. . .

CPSIA information can be obtained
at www.ICGtesting.com
Printed in the USA
LVHW052319230423
744615LV00001B/6